The Healing Room

Discovering Joy
Through the Journal

Dori Bohntinsky

*Blessings
Dori*

In-Word Bound Publishing
Castro Valley, California

The Healing Room
Copyright © 2002 by Dori Bohntinsky
All rights reserved.

Design and Printing by

Falcon Books
San Ramon, California

Cover: Original artwork by Cj Bohntinsky, May 1999

ISBN 0-9719457-0-5

FIRST EDITION

Published by
In-Word Bound Publishing
P.O. Box 20248
Castro Valley, CA 94546

PRINTED IN THE UNITED STATES OF AMERICA

*This book is dedicated to my husband and
soul mate, Chuck,
and to our beautiful daughter,
Elise Kathryn Bohntinsky.*

*It is in loving memory of our daughter,
Christen Jean (Cj) Bohntinsky
and my parents,
James and Dorothy Fraser.*

Table of Contents

Acknowledgements

I first want to acknowledge my favorite formal teachers. I had the honor to listen to most of them at seminars. I read their books. Wayne Dyer's and Deepak Chopra's writings showed me that I am a wise spiritual being having a human experience. Betty Bethards, Inner Light Foundation, taught me many practical tools for self-insight and spiritual growth (such as "cancel"). Gary Zukav, through *The Seat of the Soul*, encouraged me to face my fears.

My greatest teacher, Cj, taught me to step into the healing room by the example that she set throughout her four-month illness. When she was twelve years old, she told me that one of her greatest fears was disappointment. I told her that I believed the feeling of disappointment would be just as strong whether you looked forward to the event or worried that the event would not happen. At age fourteen, Cj was diagnosed with a rare and life threatening illness. Throughout her four-month battle and up to the moment of her going under conscious sedation, many people did not give up hope for her recovery, not Cj, not her family, friends nor many people in the medical field. However, some people were pessimistic and guarded their feelings. I discovered that sorrow and grief were just as strong for those who avoided their feelings and were cautious about developing hopes in Cj's recovery as for those who maintained faith while at the same time feeling sorrow. In fact, during the months that followed Cj's death, it seemed to me that the cautious ones experienced even greater pain and grief and took longer to heal from their sorrow. I saw the ones who were willing to touch their fears and step into the Healing Room discover a secret joy that lies within. I carried this lesson with me after Cj's death; I touched, felt, journaled and later re-read and re-wrote my most sorrowful moments. I discovered joy and I healed.

I also want to recognize two wonderful teachers who were my best friends and mentors. They were my parents. Through example they taught me to try to listen open-mindedly and to love unconditionally. They listened to my ideas. They listened quietly as I blundered. They listened as I grew. They listened as I changed my mind. They loved and listened so that my heart and soul could heal. My mother passed away from heart failure eight months after Cj died, and my father passed away six months after my mother. They are now all together on the Other Side.

At first I thought *The Healing Room* was about journaling my sorrow from the loss of our daughter, Cj. I did not realize until after I had written the final chapter that *The Healing Room* was my journey of healing made possible by the illnesses and passing of my daughter, mother and father. I have faith that they all three continue to guide me each day.

About the Author

My career as a speech pathologist began in 1976. For over two and a half decades I had worked rehabilitating the communication skills of neurologically impaired adults in acute medical, acute rehabilitation, neurorespiratory, and skilled nursing settings. As the manager of Speech Pathology and Audiology at the Alameda County Medical Center for over 20 years, I learned how to resolve a crises and more often how to prevent a problem from happening. I also have a private consulting practice and have written two workbooks, *Standard American English Pronunciation Training* and *Communicating with Pragmatics for Effective Speaking*. I developed and teach two additional courses, *Communication as a Force that Shapes You* and *Pragmatics: A Dynamic Factor in Speech and Language Evaluations*.

I have been a wife since 1971 and was blessed with two daughters: Elise in 1983 and Christen Jean (Cj) in 1985. We always lived close to my parents and often shared in care taking. When my parents were younger they often watched the girls. When they became elderly we began to watch over them.

I never dreamed that I would have to apply the knowledge, skills and compassion that I had developed as a health care worker to my daughter. Never before had any of my family members been struck with a life threatening illness, and certainly not a child. Soon after Cj's illness was diagnosed, I knew I would write a book about Cj's healing experience. It would be called *The Healing Room*. I was not sure how I would accomplish this because all my writing prior to Cj's illness had been limited to generating clinical reports, justifications or explaining factual information. I never believed I could write anything else. Throughout Cj's illness and then after her death, I kept journals of my experiences, including my feelings, sorrows, and what I was learning from each experience. I kept looking for the healing room, thinking Cj would certainly recover. At first I thought that the healing room was the hospital room, then our home, then back at the hospital, then in ICU, and finally at the memorial service.

After Cj died, I realized that the healing room was not a room at all; it was in my heart. *The Healing Room* was not about Cj's recovery, but about mine. When I wrote down my greatest moments of pain, not only from the loss of my daughter but also the loss of my mother and then father, my heart healed. After writing about a painful experience, I would relax and then I would complete my journal entry with an insight. I did not begin journaling or writing with any talents, set beliefs or understanding in mind. My ability to journal, my understanding and insights evolved as I touched my feelings and wrote.

I know everyone is encouraged to write and keep journals. I remember having assignments to write journals in high school. However, I never knew to follow each description of my experience with observations of my feelings, the lesson, my growth and then my healing. I did not discover how to journal until my own ability evolved. For several months after Cj passed away I kept wondering how I was going to write *The Healing Room*. Then I realized that it was to be a book about discovering the ability to heal from sorrow through journaling, and I had been writing it all along. It is my hope that by sharing our loss of Cj and the way I learned to journal, others will discover their own ability to journal. I hope others will no longer fear touching their pain, sorrow, and grief caused by any loss. I hope many will discover personal insights and experience the joy that follows when they enter the healing room.

Introduction

At the beginning of Cj's illness I thought the healing room was a place, a room with a large window and a beautiful view where the kind nurses, doctors, social worker and psychologist came to speak to Chuck and me about Cj's illness. I thought it was a room decorated with balloons, cards, posters, flower arrangements and banners. As Cj's illness came to an end, I began to discover that the healing room was not a room at all. The Healing Room was within me.

Cj's diagnosis forced me to face my greatest phobia—death. I was not afraid of my own death, but I feared death in general. I could not even deal with a small dead mouse, let alone walk past an open casket. Until Cj's illness, I had never experienced a life threatening illness of a loved one. I believe this was to my benefit because I did not have any precedents to follow or any preconceived notions on how to think or behave. I decided to try and understand the discovery by the ancient poet, Rumi: For every sip of sorrow there is an equal measure of joy. Also, Gary Zukav, author of *The Seat of the Soul*, wrote that every experience was a lesson for the evolution of the soul. I decided that all this must suggest that the soul feels joy each time it evolves. If everything that comes my way truly has something wonderful and powerful to teach me, then there must be a lesson in each sip of sorrow.

I decided to journal my experiences because I would need to recall specific events for my book. However, I did not realize how many sorrowful entries I would be making. Throughout

Cj's illness I kept expecting Cj to recover in the healing room, but my family and I experienced disappointment over and over again. I slowly began to touch my pain. I grieved silently or with wails and tears, and then I discovered a beautiful lesson. Following each painful moment I felt a part of myself heal. I shared my experiences and insights with the medical staff, friends and families. They all encouraged me to keep writing. I knew I could learn and integrate my greatest lesson: Healing comes from pain and sorrow if I am willing to feel my emotions and learn from the experience.

I entered the Healing Room each time I wrote down a journal entry. After a couple of months, my entries expanded beyond being a diary about the different procedures, the medication, how Cj was responding and brief comments about my feelings. I began to disclose my sorrows. I discovered that I gained greater insight into myself each time I wrote about my pain. At first, I shared my entries with family and friends as a way to keep them informed of Cj's progress and then later, to share my recovery from grief. I found that by sharing my insights, other people were also healing from their own grief. Friends and health care workers asked me to keep writing.

During Cj's illness I watched how she was a teacher to all who loved and cared for her. Many who knew her discovered what was really important to them. They learned not to take life for granted but to live each day as a wonderful blessing. Family, friends and the medical staff learned that each challenge could be viewed as an opportunity to grow. The medical staff was often awed by Cj's ability to learn about her condition and the specific care that she needed. At only fourteen years of age, she demonstrated to the doctors and nurses that mistakes are prevented and excellent care is facilitated when we take charge of our own care, as long as it does not conflict with the professional opinion of the doctor.

When Cj passed away, we did not find the books about grief very helpful. Many of the writers' opinions did not match our experiences or insights into the sorrows that followed the loss of a loved one, especially a child. Chuck, Elise and I wondered if some of these authors had actually experienced a profound loss. We read that it was normal to feel one way or another, normal to gain or lose weight, normal to cry, etc. We knew this already. One writer said to get tough because there wasn't any God. Nowhere did I read about how to use grief to discover myself. I did not find one book that encouraged us to journal our experiences to gain insights.

Several weeks after Cj passed away, we received a two-page hand-written letter from an anesthesiologist. This letter confirmed my belief that *The Healing Room* was needed. I could also recognize that by writing the letter this doctor was growing from the loss of his patient. I am sharing a part of that letter:

Although we only spent a few hours together, I feel that it was almost a lifetime . . . . As a seasoned veteran I have grown accustomed to dealing with illness, grief, shock, and can usually discuss all medical issues with patients and parents. . . . However, every once and awhile, a child comes along that truly strikes a cord with me, and despite my training and experience, their condition goes straight to my heart. . . . I admire your compassion, wisdom and humor, especially your ability to express your feelings and thoughts in such a clear and insightful way. You could show your love and caring for Cj and still be able to make the most difficult but right decision to let nature take her and allow her to seek her peaceful journey.

I wish you the strength, wisdom and love to be able to get through this part of your life. I hope that you can share your wisdom with others since you are such great teachers.

Through journaling, I entered the Healing Room often. While writing *The Healing Room*, I had to re-read all my journal entries. I discovered how far I had traveled from my early entries to the entries that I wrote months and then over a year after Cj's passing. I noticed that my writing evolved into clearer descriptions of events, circumstances and experiences. I began to describe my feelings and emotions that each painful event triggered and the insights that followed each reflection with greater ease. My insights revealed more clearly the life lessons that I needed to help me grow and heal.

I am sharing this journal of my sorrows and the insights that I discovered each time I touched my grief, in the hope that you will discover your own ability to journal. You too can write about your heartache and discover your own Healing Room. I am not encouraging you to accept my insights; mine were necessary for me to heal. I encourage you to discover your own insights and truths and heal by journaling your own pain and sorrow, regardless of your loss. May you feel joy each time a little part of you heals.

One

The Beginning

In August 1999, I read a book by Gary Zukav called *The Seat of the Soul*. I learned that each situation I encountered and my responses were necessary for the evolution and the healing of my soul. The shape of that experience, the impact of that experience and the lessons from the experience are determined by my choices.

Soon after Cj was diagnosed, I remembered a story I had heard about a Civil War family. I heard the story while visiting Gettysburg, Pennsylvania in 1997, as part of a family vacation to the East Coast. I remember being very disturbed by this story and experiencing uncontrollable tears when I visited the Civil War museum and the battlefield. When I returned home, I continued to reflect on this story and tried to learn from it. I would like to share it.

Once there was a family in Tennessee, including one son and several daughters. The father was affluent and had political influence in the state. When Tennessee entered the Civil War, the father purchased a commission for his son to keep him safe behind enemy lines. The son remained protected behind the lines during many battles.

Eventually, Union soldiers captured one of the son's friends. To save his own life the friend revealed the location of the Confederate officers. The Union soldiers attacked the officers' tents and critically injured the son. The son was brought back to his father's home. The father was distraught to find his son injured; he had been convinced that his son would return home unharmed.

The father and his wife were very devout in their faith. Also, although the father was not a formal doctor he was gifted in healing. He had helped many people in his community heal both physically and spiritually. He prayed for his son's recovery and used all of his knowledge and skills to treat his son's wounds. However, he could not save his son, and his son died a painful death.

This father became very bitter and turned against the heavens. He hated God. He was very angry and refused to feel anything. He refused to feel the pain of loss. He refused to mourn and grieve. He died years later a very hostile, angry and bitter man. His wife continued to hold onto her beliefs. However, not only did she lose her son, but also at the same time she lost the husband she had known and loved so dearly.

I remember thinking, "What a sad way to leave this earth: angry and bitter. What a wasted opportunity if life was about learning from sorrow. I would not want to wake up on the Other Side and realize I had made such a mistake — living and dying angry and bitter." When I returned home I began trying to look at life very differently. I looked for the lesson each time I went through what I thought was a difficult experience or when something simply aggravated me. I did not want to have to go through the lesson that the father went through. I began to discover that every time I used the painful situation to grow, I felt a little more joyful. I felt certain that I would never have to go through anything like that Tennessee father because I had learned the lesson in a much more practical way. I believed I had learned the lesson well, so I was sure Cj would recover.

I shared this idea with a friend soon after Cj was diagnosed. My friend sent me this e-mail:

> While I am on my morning walk each day, I listen to tapes. This morning I was listening to a tape from a set that was done in tandem with Deepak Chopra and Wayne Dyer. One part struck a cord from something you said the other day, so I thought I would pass this on to you.

> Wayne was quoting Rumi: *"I saw Grief drinking a cup of sorrow and called out, 'It tastes sweet, does it not?' 'You've caught me,' Grief answered, 'and you've ruined my business. How can I sell sorrow when you know it's a blessing?'"*

> Wayne goes on to say that EVERYTHING that comes our way has something wonderful and powerful to teach us. I know when we are going through such difficult times it is not easy to see the blessings that come from it. I hope with all my heart that you can see the blessing in the pain you are suffering now. I do not even pretend to know what you are going through, but I hope today is a good day for you, your family and especially Cj.

> My thoughts are with you, my friend. I love you.

I had always heard that God would not give us a burden greater than we could handle. I felt very fortunate to have heard the story about the bitter Confederate father and had begun to discover the lessons that arise from irritating situations. I knew I had a choice. I could either become angry at the unfair tragedy that had hit my family, or I could look for that blessing that came with each cup of sorrow.

TWO

Cj's Illness

Cj had been a Castro Valley High School Freshman for two weeks when she was diagnosed on September 17, 1999, with Myelodysplastic Syndrome (MDS). MDS is a rare form of leukemia whereby the bone marrow quits making any blood (white blood cells, red blood cells and platelets). Since her body did not have white blood cells, Cj did not have an immune system. She received most of her medical care at Kaiser Permanente in Oakland, which specializes in children with cancer and blood disorders, and her final care at Children's Hospital in Oakland.

Only about one in six million people get MDS, so very little is known about treating this disease. The medical protocol was experimental. After receiving blood transfusions and platelets (blood cells that make the blood clot), Cj had surgery to have a tube (Broviac) placed next to her heart. This allowed for future transfusions and the medications to go directly into the tube instead of having an I.V. and injections all the time. The protocol consisted of three rounds of chemotherapy over a period of months and then a bone marrow transplant in late January if there was a bone marrow match. A month after Cj's diagnosis, the doctors discovered that I was Cj's match for bone marrow. This was extremely rare that a parent would be a match, about one chance in 500.

Because Cj's body did not make blood, she required over a hundred blood transfusions during the treatment period. Her body required two types of blood transfusions: Red blood transfusions, needed to provide oxygen to the body, and transfusions of platelets. Without these transfusions, Cj would not have survived beyond September. She said that one of her greatest disappointments was that she would no longer be able to donate blood or bone marrow to help other people. I realized how important regular donors are, especially for rare blood types and bone marrow. Cj's blood type (A-) was rare, and there were times that the hospital had to wait for blood. Once platelets were flown all the way from Omaha, Nebraska to Oakland in order to prepare Cj for a surgical procedure.

While in the hospital, Cj began getting involved with community organizations. She became an honoree for Team in Training, an organization that raises money for the Leukemia Society of America. Cj cut her hair off before she had chemotherapy and donated her twelve-inch curly locks to Locks of Love, an organization that provides hairpieces to financially disadvantaged children who suffer medical hair loss from chemotherapy or diseases that cause hair to permanently fall out. Cj wasn't interested in a hairpiece. She didn't mind being bald.

Every time Cj went to the hospital I decorated her room with posters, pictures of the family, artificial flowers (because she was not allowed real flowers due to the lack of an immune system), special gifts and cards. I included decorations for each holiday season. Each time I decorated, the hospital staff said no one had a room decorated like Cj's and many of the nurses took their breaks in her room. It did not make sense to me that parents did not decorate their children's rooms.

I maintained hope for Cj's recovery by using a variety of alternative therapies. Cj loved acupressure, especially on her feet. I would massage her feet every day and would talk about what part of the body was being stimulated. I used aromatherapy and essential oils, especially peppermint for nausea and lavender for relaxation. Cj loved her meditative music. She took her CD player with her for all procedures that required conscious sedation, such as the multiple spinal taps that were necessary to determine if her bone marrow had begun to develop blood cells. I put her music on for her every night before leaving the hospital. Cj loved her crystals. One day the social worker told me that she took some of her stones up to show Cj and was humbled by Cj's collection of healing stones. Cj loved art therapy. She created beautiful tiny sculptures out of clay and gave one to Elise, Chuck, the social worker and me. Chuck read aloud to her, and she loved the Harry Potter books. The medical staff, especially the social worker, said they had never seen a family deal with a life threatening illness in this way.

Cj was admitted back into the hospital on Christmas Eve due to an infection and remained in the hospital for the final month of her life. She had developed a sinus infection from a wisdom tooth coming in and then pneumonia. Cj had no immune system to fight the infection. She was in the hospital during the 2000-millenium celebration and had a great view of the San Francisco fireworks from her tenth-story window.

After complications from sinus surgery, Cj was transferred to the Intensive Care Unit (ICU) at Children's Hospital. There Chuck and I saw many parents facing the challenges of having very ill children. I realized that we were not the only parents suffering from the severe illness of a child, many families were. Everyone at Children's Hospital was either an ill or injured child, a family member or an employee.

On Saturday, January 15, Cj gave her permission to be sedated and put onto a breathing machine (ventilator) to help her lungs. I was not there that morning. Chuck told me that Cj made the doctors assure her that they would wake her up when her lungs were better. When Monday came, Cj's lungs were weaker. That evening I whispered to Cj, "I know this is really hard for you, and you can go if you really want to." However, I also told her that if she stayed she could get straight F's in high school, and I would not get upset. I am sure she knew that I was not ready to let her go. By the 18th, I felt the terror of realization that Cj was not getting better and that I would lose her. When I got home that night, Chuck, Elise and I wept in each other's arms and asked for strength.

On January 19, I returned to the hospital, once again hopeful for Cj's recovery. There she was sedated on a ventilator, being rocked in a special bed and wearing Attends (adult diapers). Still, I felt so certain that she would be all right. I knew that beautiful lessons could come from sorrow. I had lived these lessons for the past four months. I did not need Cj to die to convince me that joy can come from sorrow. I kept telling God that I knew the lesson. I did not have to experience the loss, and others did not need to suffer any more sorrow either. I had seen little miracles throughout her illness. I prayed, "God, you showed me so many miracles over the past four months and told me there would be a miracle. It cannot get any worse so where is my miracle?" A gentle thought entered my mind. "Are you sure you know what the miracle is or do you have it backwards? Is it her staying or is it her going home?" It was then that I realized that I had to do the ultimate lab work. If I was going to write *The Healing Room*, then I had to heal. I had to face my greatest fear, my greatest phobia — the death of a loved one. I could only develop a full understanding of loss if I experienced mankind's greatest loss, the loss of our child. I could not learn everything from my books. I had to do the lab work. I wept and told Cj that now I understood and that she could go home.

Cj passed away on January 20, 2000 at 8:30 p.m. during the height of the first full lunar eclipse of 2000. Many who knew Cj try to take solace in her death by thinking about what her life and her passing meant to them. Having had shots and surgical procedures, Cj said, "The fear in anticipation was always worse than the actual event." The fear and anticipation of Cj's passing caused me my greatest anguish. We all witnessed Cj's passing which was beautiful and serene; we felt grief but not anguish. I even felt awe and a great love for all mankind.

I felt blessed throughout the whole process of Cj's illness and death. I often spent at least five hours a day with Cj when she was in the hospital, and we had some very beautiful talks. However, the two times she was discharged from the hospital following chemotherapy, she took off with her sister, Elise. Chuck and I were left alone together while Cj went right back to being a teenager and having a good time. In the hospital, we talked about things that touched our souls. I told people that Cj would be okay because she was my teacher and I needed her. When Cj passed away I wondered how she could have been my teacher because I did most of the talking. A gentle thought came to me, "I did the talking, but she was the one who asked me the questions."

Three

Meet Cj

I was sharing entries from *The Healing Room* with a friend when she asked me to write about Cj because she wanted to get to know her better. I suddenly realized that while I had learned to journal my experiences and feelings, I lacked words when it came to describing Cj. As a parent, I am too close to her. I knew her for over fourteen years. There are no adequate words to describe her personality, her joys, her sorrows, her pranks, her gifts, her problems, her generosity, her wisdom nor her innocence. No, I had no words to describe Cj, but others did. Cj had written about herself. She had written a poem in school the week before she was diagnosed with MDS. She also wrote an autobiography as a "home school" assignment while in the hospital. A good friend of Elise's was the high school newspaper editor. She knew Cj and wrote about her. I know writing this article helped Elise's friend to heal. It also helped the high school to heal. Her editorial is called, "A Tribute to Cj."

Cj wrote this poem the first week of high school as a freshman. It was the last assignment she ever completed for the high school.

Christen
Unique, giving, out going, considerate
Daughter of the world
Lover of the written word
   all music
   water falling from the sky
Who feels the hurt in others eyes
   a good book could cure a bad day
   that everyone is important
Who needs to express herself
   to be excused from doing the dishes
   to listen to music everyday
Who fears what she can't see
   being alone
   the wrath of others
Who gives all she can
   time to children
   friendship to those who are deserving
Who would like to see World Hunger end
   the castles of Scotland
   a female President
Resident of this reality
   Bohntinsky 9/9/99

Cj wrote the following autobiography as an assignment for home (hospital) school about one month after being diagnosed with MDS. It was the first time she ever focused so much on illness.

October 1999

My entire life I have had problems with my health. I developed asthma shortly after I was born. As an infant I had ear infections. At age nine I started getting warts on my feet. During middle school it seems I was constantly missing school due to a cold or the flu. In the last few months, I have been diagnosed with a serious illness known as Myelodysplastic Syndrome (MDS).

Asthma has been part of my life as long as I can remember. I had my first asthma attack when I was about one and a half. In the first five years of my life I had three asthma attacks that sent me to the hospital for several nights. My last severe asthma attack was when I was five years old. I was in the hospital for a week. I remember getting a pass for Thanksgiving. I wore a purple and pink dress to my grandparents' house. All my mother's family was there. My parents and I learned to control my asthma with medication. I have also outgrown it a little.

When I was nine I had this blister on my foot that wouldn't go away. After a couple of months the blister started to look like a wart. My parents and I decided not to do any thing about it for a couple of years. When I was eleven I had about seven warts on my feet. They were starting to bother me and bleed. My mom took me to a dermatologist. I remember that at one time I had thirteen warts on my feet. They didn't hurt but I was embarrassed about the way my feet looked. I still have two warts on my feet but I don't really care.

In middle school it seemed like I would get sick a lot more than most of the other kids at my school. I would miss school at about an average of two days a month. It seemed like I was always sick. Although I got the flu shot every year because of my asthma, it seemed I'd get some kind of flu that caused me to miss school.

After the first week of high school I got sick. My parents thought it was the flu. On Saturday I had a temperature of one hundred and two and an excruciating headache. During that week in September I started to get paler and paler. Thursday morning I woke up with a bruise under my eye. My mom called the hospital that morning from her work. She told the nurse about my symptoms. I went to see the doctor that afternoon.

The doctor said that I might have mono but she didn't think it was that serious. My mom and I walked half a block to the lab. They drew blood and did a test called a cut test. A cut test is when they make a small shallow cut on your arm. Then they watch to see how long it bleeds. After that my mom and I walked back to our car which was in the hospital parking lot.

That night a doctor from Hayward Kaiser called and said I needed to come in right away. My parents, my sister and I went over to Kaiser quickly. We had been at Hayward about thirty minutes when they told us to go to Oakland. They said Oakland had a better hematology ward and they had a bed available. We went straight to admitting at Oakland. It was about eleven forty when we got there, the women from admitting asked if we could wait until midnight to admit me. We waited because it had some thing to do with the shift change. I didn't understand.

Once we got to the pediatric floor I had an I.V. put in my arm. It took four tries to put the I.V. in, and that was one of the most painful things I have had done to me so far. Then I got a platelet transfusion. Later I got several red blood cell transfusions.

The doctors told my parents that I either had aplastic ane-mia or leukemia. They did some tests and found out I had aplastic anemia. Two out of one million people get aplastic anemia. The doctors soon found that I had myelodysplastic syndrome (MDS) which one third of the people with aplastic anemia get, or one out of six million people. I think I have dealt with having a serious illness well. My body is responding well to the treatments. I can't wait until this is all a memory.

This front-page editorial appeared in the Castro Valley High School newspaper on February 11, 2000. It was written by the school's newspaper editor, Elise's good friend, Helen.

A Tribute to Cj

She was born Christen Jean Bohntinsky but to those of us who knew her, loved her and cherished her, she was always Cj. She was Cj with the hair that begged to be pulled, Cj with gigantic boots, Cj with the smile for everyone.

Robert Frost wrote, "Nature's first green is gold. Her hardest hue to hold. Nothing gold can stay." Cj was pure gold. For 14 brief years she shone and sparkled, a brilliant star shedding its light into even the darkest of souls. But like the brightest of stars in the galaxy, she burned with so much passion for life that she had to go home early. Her physical body is gone, but her spirit is intransient and remains within all of us who knew her. Her "goldness" is something that defies Frost's ideology, for Cj will live on eternally: her courage, her laughter, her music, and her individuality.

It would be misleading to say that Cj was a saint, one who was a pure and blameless model angel. She was anything but. Cj was human, a child. She had all the characteristics of a young girl, including mischievousness, a love for fun, and spontaneity, but she was also a helper and a nurturer.

Whether it was a loving smile or a hand offered in friend-ship, Cj always looked for ways to make others' lives better. Her friends remember water fights with water bot-tles on a hot day, but her grandfather remembers her de-termination in painting their fence when she already lacked the energy to do everyday things. This was before anyone ever thought she was sick. By her actions Cj taught us how to live, with kindness, love, courage and water fights.

My favorite memory of Cj is almost ludicrous in its silli-ness. It was the summer of my sophomore year, and Cj's sister (my best friend Elise) and I were signing up for sum-mer school at Chabot. Afterwards with Elise at the wheel, Mrs. Bohntinsky, Cj and I were hanging on for dear life. As Elise made a quick, casual U-turn, a gigantic semi-truck came bearing down on us, horns blaring. The four of us did what any normal, rational human would do, we screamed. Eventually, though, Elise, Cj, and I dis-solved into hysterical laughter. There was such a feeling of LIFE in the air, a palpable quality of energy and youth. That liveliness was a constant in Cj, a precious trait that made her all the more endearing. In her short life she had more life and more vitality in her than most people would accumulate over a lifetime.

Cj, even though I cannot see her anymore, if I strain to lis-ten, I can still hear her laughter and the click of the boots on the pavement. You were wrong, Mr. Robert Frost. Some gold does stay.

Four

The Cj Chronicles

9/16/99 - 1/19/2000

Chuck wrote short entries about Cj and her illness almost daily. I found these invaluable when I wanted to remember when a specific incident happened and I will always be thankful that we both took the time to write. While my memories have faded, I can always look back at the chronicles when I want to remember something about the illness. What I found to be interesting, though, was that I journaled much less than Chuck during Cj's illness. However, my initial entries shared a limited amount of information regarding the specifics of Cj's illness and focused more on how Cj was doing and how I was perceiving each situation. I also noticed that it did not take long before I began to include personal insights into myself after journaling about the medical events.

I journaled more after Cj passed away, and I believe I healed from my tragic loss. When I read a draft of *The Healing Room* about twenty months after Cj's death I noticed that Chuck stopped journaling the day before Cj passed away. I read what he wrote on January 19, and realized that his final entry seemed to reveal where he still was. It was as if time had stopped for him. He still seemed to miss her every moment. When I would ask him if he had any sense of personal insight around our loss he would say, "No." A day rarely went by that he did not say, "I miss Cj." I continued to journal my pain and sorrows. Each time I journaled, I discovered an insight and then experienced a personal joy. I felt myself heal a little bit more.

The CJ Chronicles are short entries that Chuck and I made almost day-by-day during Cj's illness. Chuck made his entries almost daily into his small hand-held computer (a Palm Pilot) up to the day before Cj passed away. I wrote in my journal or on the computer. I have intertwined my early short entries with Chuck's.

Chuck:

9/16/99 - Cj checked in @ 10:00 p.m. at Hayward Kaiser. At 12:00 checked into 916A in Oakland Kaiser.

9/17 - Cj wants book on Buddhism, batteries, toothbrush, and clothes. Talked with Dr. Month.

9/18 - Most of family visited. Cj is getting some "color" due to transfusions.

Dori:

9/18/99 - On Thursday, September 16, I took Cj to Kaiser Hospital because she had been sick all week with flu-like symptoms. That evening (9:30) we received a call to bring her to the hospital due to low platelets and anemia. On Friday we learned that she has aplastic anemia – a serious condition. The bone marrow stopped making blood. It is idiopathic (of unknown cause). It is most likely from a virus. Her hemoglobin was 3 (normal is 12 – 15). Today she had her fifth blood transfusion. She has color and is chipper. This is a lesson in true sorrow. We will know the course of treatment next Thursday. She may have a bone marrow transplant if Elise is a match (25% chance). Otherwise, a medicinal approach will be necessary to get her bone marrow working. Right now the bone marrow is not making white blood cells; therefore, Cj does not have an immune system. The prognosis is hopeful. However, recovery will be slow.

I feel sorrow. I mourn Cj's loss of health. I mourn the unknown. I know this is mine to go through. This is each of ours to go through in our own way. It is an individual lesson for each of us. I cry. I do hurt. It is not a stabbing pain in the chest, but in my mind.

Chuck:

9/24 - Dori & I learning Broviac care (the tube that goes into her chest). Cj is to come home for weekend. Chemotherapy to start Monday — Chuck worried.

9/25, 26 - Good weekend all considered — Cj slept well, sore from surgery & sore throat. Her friend Andrea visited on Sunday afternoon. Elise, Andrea and (great-uncle) John Short watched as Dori cut Cj's hair.

9/27 - Checked back into room 920 @ 9:15 am. Cj is very tired and pensive.

Dori:

9/27 - A lot has happened since the 19th. Cj has myelodysplastic syndrome according to the bone marrow biopsy. This means that the blood cells that are being produced look different, and there is chromosome involvement. There are about 10% blasts. These blasts (cancer producing cells) can develop (will) into leukemia if not treated. I have been preparing for this. My heart goes from pain to feelings of hope and peace. Cj's illness is impacting so many people.

I receive strength through meditation. Right now it is hard to find a quiet place. However, I can meditate and pray anywhere with any sounds around. I am learning to be meditative and be in the moment. One of my sisters, Charlee, said the Bible says, "God's words guide me like a lantern guides my steps." We realized that in those days an oil lantern only guided a few steps at a time. I can only go through this experience one step at a time in order to stay focused. I hear messages when my mind is clear. I feel less pain when my mind is clear. I can listen to a crying sick baby in peace when my mind is clear.

At times, I forget to tune into my energy, especially when feeling apprehensive. Decisions will need to be made. Are these for me to decide? Decisions do not need to be made right away. We may need to think about it and be tuned into our intuition. Then decisions are easier to make. I also am learning to give up control. Many will be helping Cj; they are her servants and the servants of the Divine.

Chuck:

9/28 - Cj is feeling better and handling chemotherapy well — Chuck, Anu, Grandmom visited. Moved to 10th floor isolation unit ... very nice. Elise visited in evening — Cj happy to spend time with her. Chuck and Dori went to Valerian Cafe for dinner. Marge and Bill (Cj's godparents) found us and sat with us while we ate ... nice.

10/2 - Brought Cj home. Quiet day. Cj seems ok.

Dori:

10/2 - I am working to stay in the now. A Catholic friend shared words from a Buddhist Monk, "Not yesterday, not tomorrow, now." My pain moves in and out. I had laryngitis for two days and had to speak less and listen. This is hard for me. I thought I was becoming quieter, but the laryngitis showed me how much I depend on speaking. When I am silent I can tune into the messages from others and those from my intuition (or guiding voice).

Chuck:

10/3 - Quiet day at home — Dori's parents (Frasers) visited for short time.

10/4-6 - Cj at home — scared to sleep in bed and slept with Dori on Tuesday night. On 10/5 braces removed. Very tired — Cj says she is ready to return to hospital.

10/7 - Checked into hospital — had 102 temperature. Antibiotics started along with chemotherapy.

Dori:

10/7 - I am back in the hospital with Cj. She will start her second five days of chemotherapy. I had to hold back tears when I entered her room. Staying centered keeps me strong. Cj has a temperature and does not feel well. She is short with me, and I do not blame her. This is a lesson in being loving and neutral and to serve her when I am needed.

Chuck:

10/8-11 - Chemo and antibiotics. Cj sick—vomiting & diaharrea. Lost hair. Spent weekend at hospital — Chuck usually arrives between 9 and 10 a.m. and Dori stays until 11 p.m. Cj had spinal tap on 11th and did ok. Temperature spikes up to 103.

Dori:

10/10 - I gave Cj a buzz cut as she requested. Yesterday, she was literally pulling out her hair and laughing. Her hair cut took quite awhile with Chuck's beard trimmer. Cj has an infection and will have to stay in the hospital for about a month.

10/11 - This is Cj's last day of chemotherapy for round one. Right now she is getting a spinal tap. I am so peaceful in the hospital with Cj. It is a very meditative experience. I feel so surrounded by love. Few of us really know what love is. It is the opposite of hate. We know hate but love often eludes us. Love is not physical, as we so often mistake it. The closest feeling is joy. Joy for no reason. Rejoice. Rejoice in all things, especially health.

Chuck:

10/12 - Cj was due to come home but has an infection. Once antibiotics are started she must remain in hospital until white blood counts are up. Could be many months? Amphotericin causes Cj major chills at 90 minutes. Shots of Demerol controls chills. Demerol causing vomiting within 5 minutes. Note: Impenium was discontinued (10/18?) — stopped nausea and reaction to Demerol.

10/13 - Started G-CSF shots, a medication to kick-start development of white blood cells.

Dori:

10/14 - I am sitting here at work looking at my timesheet and am again torn between documenting exact times and any eight hours. What is my dilemma? What is this timesheet? I allow my staff to write a consistent time but do not allow myself. As a manager, I do not even have to according to the law. However, I believe it is unethical to write the wrong time. Ethics is a judgement. What is ethical in one society or group is not in another. "To thine own self be true." I have worked less hard and that has been OK with me. The timesheet is up to me. It does not matter. It is so challenging though. There must be a lesson.

What is work? It is serving others. Is there really such a thing as work? It is a presence doing different things at different places. "Work" versus "play" is a judgement. "How long is my presence in my office?" That is what is judged. I do not need to bring judgement upon myself regarding this ignorant value. I therefore release the power this timesheet has had over me. It is so hard to balance work with Cj's illness.

Chuck:

10/15 - Talked with Dr. Month — Dori is close enough match for Cj's bone marrow transplant. Need to call and meet with Dr. Horn at UCSF. Went to dinner with Marge & Bill after their visit. Nice.

10/16,17 - Uneventful weekend. Nice meditative time with Cj. Still sick but good spirits.

10/18 - Chuck had business planning meetings; got to hospital about 6:00 p.m. Dori comes to hospital about 4:00 p.m. each weekday and stays until 10 p.m. or later.

10/19 - Chuck took day off to be at hospital; Cj Still sick. Nice time with Cj.

10/20 - Met with Dr. Horn @ UCSF. Very difficult meeting — Dori broke down — Chuck too. Told the chances are high of losing her. Very tough day.

10/21 - Chuck returned to work for Business Planning. Talked to Krista on phone regarding diagnosis — tears. Cj had "good day" but started period early — lots of clots. Not nauseous and no temp spikes. Had sonogram — gall stones only abnormality. Cj gave me big hug when I arrived at hospital … had to hide tears.

10/22 - Tough day @ work — finished business planning. Talked to my boss, Cherie. She was very upset. Talked to

Debbie & Jeff ... tears. Cj received platelets in early a.m. Menstrual period heavy and concerned about Broviac site infection.

Dori:

10/22 - Last Friday we found out that I am a match for Cj's bone marrow. It is a miracle. On Wednesday, 10/20, Chuck and I went to the University of California in San Francisco (UCSF) for a consultation. It was a very "sobering" and "sorrowful" experience to read Dr. Month's letter to Dr. Horn. Maybe I did not fully realize, or accept, the seriousness of Cj's condition. According to Dr. Month, though, Cj is doing better than many children who have had two rounds of chemotherapy. Wednesday was a very sorrowful day and I mourned. It was like re-living the diagnosis all over again. It was hard to hold back tears. I cried driving home and in the bathroom. I recalled crying at that same spot in the bathroom once before due to the canyon in front of our home being filled in with dirt in order for a road and the creation of lots for homes. I have come far since then.

Cj did not throw up yesterday. A sonogram showed the organs are fine. However, she has gallstones. These are not a concern as long as they do not bother her. I feel like I have not had time to meditate. However, I feel at peace going to work and then to Oakland Kaiser, then home to bed. I am learning to be meditative; to silence my mind during activities. I am learning to live in the moment. By living in the moment and silencing my mind I am more aware of my intuition and what I like to call little miracles. I used to operate on reasoning. Now I am learning to use intuition and "see" the Guidance.

Chuck:

10/23 - I arrived about 9:15 a.m. Cj sleeping from Benadryl. Started Ampho and Cj got chills. Demerol calmed her.

10/24-31 - Medicines include Amphotericin B, Vancomycin Hydrochloride, Tobramycin Sulfate, Ceftazidime Sodium/Dextrose-WA2, and Hyperal. Started running temperature up to 103 from Wednesday through Sunday while Ampho being given. On Tuesday night the junction into Broviac cracked — possible link to infection/temperature …scary for Cj to wake up to blood. Also in menstrual period all week, lots of bleeding and clots. Started new birth control pills. Much higher dosage of Estrogen. Talked to Dr. Month on Thursday — bone marrow transplant in January now part of protocol. SCARED (Chuck).

Dori:

11/05 - Cj has been in the hospital for one month. Her spirits remain high, and the nursing staff and doctors adore her. A friend of mine came by my work yesterday. She said she has a black spot on her lung. We must all accept responsibility for our part in the "cause/effect." When we blame others for our condition our energy goes down. When we deny feelings, our energy goes down.

Today I learned that I do fear death; we all do. It is part of the human experience. I also realized that I do worry. I just did not know what it felt like. My supervisor has been a good teacher regarding this. I thought I feared authority. It's really that I worry around authority. My energy goes low when I am criticized. It is authority that can criticize me. I stay pretty up when Cj or Chuck criticizes me, but even then my energy goes low for a short time. It is this low energy, this sense of loss that I fear. However, I criticize; therefore I am criticized. As I discover how to take criticism joyfully, appreciating the lesson that Life is sending me, I will equally grow in my ability to criticize. Criticism does not need to be a judgement. When it is a judgement I will learn to take it as it is — an opinion.

Chuck:

11/1-10 - Cj's "counts" returning — platelets still very low, white blood count is up to 30K. Still in period, clots. Dr. Month said there are no chromosomal problems with last bone marrow test. Cj discharged on 11/10, Wednesday evening.

11/11-21 - Cj at home. Wanted to go to San Francisco Zoo. Went on Saturday (11/13), fun and Cj liked the wheelchair but got pretty tired. On Monday, Dori drew Cj's blood for a blood test and drove blood to lab.

11/28 - 12/23 - At home. Getting Ampho & blood on Monday, Wednesday, and Friday. Occasionally sleeping with Mom & Dad. Very lethargic most of the time. Skin peeling from palms of hands and soles of feet.

12/20/99 - Cj with Dori in hospital waiting for platelets after Amphotericin. Very sick with mouth sores, wisdom tooth, low counts. Taking Septra, penicillin, potassium, and G-CSF shots. Slept with us in waterbed last night.

12/24 - Very frustrating news — Cj back in hospital due to temperature of 102.2. Jennifer (nurse) and Dr. Campbell said she would have to stay. Cj & Dad cried — very disappointed. All Cj wanted was to be home for Christmas.

12/24-1/11/2000 - Cj in hospital with sinus problems. On PCA Morphine constantly (Patient-Controlled-Dosage machine). Depressed and cranky, not very responsive and bothered by noise and lights. Started period again, getting lots of platelets and blood transfusions. Antibiotics are constant along with Hyperal. Tough times right now. Counts are low and not moving. G-CSF shots were useless while at home due to misunderstanding. Cj has received 15 productive shots. Last night (1-10-2000) she had another CT scan and chest x-ray.

Very tearful and difficult for her to wait for tests ... two poles, and wheelchair handled by Chuck and Dori.

1/13/2000 -

- 10:00a.m. — Looks to be a very tough day. Abdominal pain, another Ultra sound is due — Cj very upset. Surgery this afternoon for sinus but very low platelets (concerned because the count is 19,000 and 40,000 is minimum for safe surgery). Needs blood and platelet transfusion plus all antibiotics.

- 5:00p.m. — Cj had ultra sound, chest x-ray and CT Scan in a.m. Had to drink 2 cups of barium for CT scan. Doctor Organ and Orloff very concerned regarding stomach pain. Nothing conclusive — Orloff said life threatening. Chuck & Dori numb ... too much. Surgery for sinus started at 2:30p.m. with Dr. Cruz. Said it went ok — no major bleeding. Took out some polyps and said there was some "chronic" infection but no puss due to no white blood cells. Cj in much pain. Chuck could not bear to see her suffering ... had to go to cafeteria for coffee.

- 5:00p.m. - 9:30p.m. — Cj choking on swallowed blood draining from sinus cavity — very concerned. At 9:30 moved to ICU @ Children's Hospital in Oakland. Chuck came home, Dori stayed and will call.

1/14 - Took Cj to Children's. Good care but tough day on Friday — lung issues, stomach infection (typhlitis). Chuck stayed until 9:00, Dori until 11:00 p.m.

1/15 - Saturday ... Chuck arrived and talked with Cj about need for ventilator until her lungs strengthen. Helped her go to bathroom. Doctors put her under general at 10:50 a.m. to put in breathing tube. Cj said I did not have to stay in to watch. She said, "I don't think you can take this." Chuck called Elise. Dori on her way. Chuck talked to doctor — her stomach not bothering her as much. Chuck put on CD music: Medicine Woman. I know she can hear this and feel my thoughts. The ICU nurse, LuAnne talking to Cj and telling her how well she is doing. My thoughts: Looking at my daughter, so beautiful and important to me... to us. She is relaxing for the first time in days. Eyes half-open white fuzzy hair shimmering. I want to take away all her pain. She handles it so courageously.

- Dr. Orloff & Dr. Michaelson: They are responsible for worrying.

- 1:30p.m. — Nurse Luanne said the pulmonary biopsy procedure went well. Lower right lobe has infection, and cultures will help determine antibiotic.

1/16/2000 - Susan is nurse. Cj is still under. Uneventful night — temp spike with ampho. Cj looks like a large beautiful baby. Temp about 102 when we arrived @ 11:00 a.m. Slight swelling in hands and face. Dr. talked to us — more fluids in body (2 liters), no activity and protein imbalance. They will keep her under sedation through tonight because breathing machine is supplying O2 at 53 (normal air is 40). Cj would have to work too hard to keep her oxygen saturation level up if taken off the ventilator.

1/17/2000 - Cj sedated on ventilator. Lungs causing concern so they put her on a different machine. She may be intubated for long time — weeks? Still having menstrual hemorrhaging with very large clots. Getting progesterone, which tricks the body into thinking it's pregnant. Vitals: heart rate = 140, respiration = 25, blood pressure = 110/60/75, Oxygen saturation = 95 at 66 on ventilator.

Luanne is the nurse during day. Gave lasix. Ordered a different bed that rocks to help pneumonia.

1/18/2000 - Worked in Rancho Cordova. Met w/ Krista, Bonny, Rich, and David and told them of desperate situation. Arrived @ Children's 3:00p.m. and talked with Dr. Month — very little chance for recovery. Aspirgillis fungal virus is pervasive in lungs, sinus, blood. Dori arrived about 4 p.m. We talked to Cj and each other. Dr. Month said it could happen quickly.

1/19/2000 - Thoughts: I already miss Cj. She is such a beautiful person … so caring of us. I will miss her every moment for the rest of my life.

Five

Good Morning E-mail

On weekends, Chuck and I often sent e-mails to family, friends and work colleagues to keep them informed of Cj's condition. Friends said that these e-mails helped them cope with their anxieties over Cj's illness. Writing the initial e-mails helped us because we would sit down and organize the events that had happened during the week. We would reflect on what had happened, the present situation and what we needed to do next. Interestingly, when I read this e-mail a year later, I noticed that I had not shared my feelings nor my insights.

10/10/99

A pleasant Sunday morning to you all, and thank you for your thoughts and prayers. Cj has been a role model for dealing with illness. She has a great attitude and is handling everything amazingly well. Her condition is serious, but we all believe that she will recover. Her diagnosis is officially known as Myelodysplastic Syndrome . . . a form of Leukemia known as Oligoblastic Leukemia. It is a disorder characterized by low blood counts and a bone marrow that typically has an increasing number of "blasts" (cancerous cells).

This disorder is treated with very aggressive chemotherapy. Cj is in the second phase of the first round of chemotherapy.

There will be three rounds spaced months apart. So far she is handling the chemotherapy well. She has had temperature spikes up to 104 degrees from an infection (the doctors assure us this is typical, although serious). Infection is their major concern, and it will be watched very carefully for the next several months. Cj will be done with this phase of chemotherapy on Monday, but since she has had an infection, she will be staying in the hospital for a while longer. She could potentially be in the hospital for many months. After this first round, Cj will be starting "drug" therapy via shots. The intent is to kick-start her immune system, which happens in about 80% of people going through this. She will start the second round of chemotherapy when her system starts producing normal cells.

Cj is in great spirits. She has the nurses and doctors amazed at how well she is handling all this. Several of the nurses have told Chuck and me that they have never seen anyone with a better attitude. For example, Cj was laughing yesterday at being able to pull out her hair. She said, "This place is making me so crazy that I am pulling my hair out." Then she reached to her head and pulled out clumps of hair. She actually seems to be enjoying her changing appearance.

Thanks again for all your positive energy.

Love Chuck, Dori, Elise, and Cj

Six

An E-Mail Update

Since mid October, Chuck, Elise and I had helped Cj through the side effects of chemotherapy. Chuck and I had both been journaling, not to others but for ourselves. I did not write any formal e-mails between early November and early December. I had been very busy taking Cj back and forth to the hospital for preventative treatments. I continued working, and I was preparing our home for the holidays. I finally sat down one Saturday and wrote this e-mail to our family, friends and work colleagues. Some of this information was covered previously in the Introduction or in the chapter about Cj's illness because, at the time, I pulled information from those entries to write this e-mail. I chose to leave this e-mail in its original form and not remove the redundant information. I noticed that in this e-mail I was beginning to share more personal insights about myself.

12/4/99

Dear Friends and Family,

Thank you for your prayers and wishes for well-being and continued concern for Cj's recovery. She continues to be a wonderful source of strength for all of us. She finished round two of three rounds of chemotherapy the Saturday after

Thanksgiving. She chose to be in the hospital during Thanksgiving in order to be home for Christmas.

She goes to the hospital every Monday, Wednesday and Friday to have an antibiotic infused through the Broviac (the central line in her chest). This infusion takes about five hours to complete if all goes smoothly (like the pharmacy sending up the medication in a timely manner). We are hoping that she will no longer have to receive this infusion once she has an immune system. The oncologists told us that this is the first time that they are doing this procedure for a patient before an infection. Cj has remained out of the hospital following this second round of chemotherapy because she has not yet gotten a fever. The doctors continue to be very pleased with Cj's ability to resist getting infections. We believe it is due to the fact that a loving staff, friends, family and the healing energy of God surround her. Her strong spirit, sense of humor, and ability to recognize and be honest about her feelings has also contributed to her healing.

Cj is certainly a teacher by helping me to discover what is really important to me. She has taught me not to take life for granted, but to live each day as a wonderful blessing. I have learned how blessed my family really is. I am learning to view each challenge as the opportunity to grow as a person. Since this second round of chemotherapy, Cj has shown me that the greatest fear really is fear itself. When I trust that all things are for a purpose, I gain the ability to see the miracles that surround us daily. The medical staff is often awed by Cj's knowledge about her condition and the specific care that she needs. Cj knows that she is in charge of her own care whenever it does not conflict with the professional opinion of the doctor.

Cj is even getting involved with community organizations. She has become an honoree for Team in Training, an organization that raises money for the Leukemia Society of America. Non-athletic individuals are sponsored to bike or run/walk official marathons all over the country. Once Cj recovers from her bone marrow transplant, she will attend some of the training sessions and kick off events to inspire the participants to finish the race.

Cj also donated her twelve-inch curly locks to Locks of Love. She cut them off before she had chemotherapy. This organization provides hairpieces to financially disadvantaged children who suffer medical hair loss from chemotherapy or alopecia areata, a disease that causes hair to permanently fall out. Cj isn't interested in a hairpiece or even hats. She doesn't mind being bald.

In January, Cj will undergo chemotherapy once more and have the bone marrow transplant. The wonderful miracle is that I am her donor. Cj will be at the University of California San Francisco Medical Center for at least six to eight weeks. I believe that this will be Cj's time for final healing. A stated risk of the transplant is that Cj could acquire medical conditions in the future from my genes if she has a predisposition towards these conditions. However, I believe that since Cj is having the transplant to receive my good cells, she will be healthier than she has ever been because I am blessed with good health.

We wish you all well during this holiday season. Thank you again for all your powerful prayers; God does work miracles. As we say good-bye to the 1900's may we all look towards a new millennium where mankind is bonded in spirit.

Seven

The Error

One of Chuck's colleagues offered to read and edit a draft of *The Healing Room*. We got together about a month later, which happened to be a week after the tragic implosion of the World Trade Center in September 2001. We met for dinner to discuss her comments and to answer questions she had about the book. Later on in our conversation, I felt comfortable enough to disclose information that I had chosen not to include in the book. I shared that during Cj's illness I had to face great fears and sorrows, and I revealed one of my greatest ones to her. I revealed the error. She asked why I had not included this experience in the book. I told her it was too personal and too painful an experience to share. However, what I really wanted to say was that the error carried with it an almost overwhelming "what if someone found out this about me?" Before leaving, she apologized for not returning the manuscript sooner. Then she said, "I finished reading it after the tragedy of the World Trade Center. I was devastated and depressed because of the attack. When I finished reading the manuscript a part of me healed." She began to journal.

Later, while I was re-editing the book, I realized that I was not doing what I believed to be so important in healing. I was not sharing my pain in the manner that I knew was necessary for me to heal. I realized that including the error was not only important for encouraging others to touch their most fearful pain, but it would help my wound heal. I knew this entry was in my journal, but I had conveniently decided to leave it out. I did not want the world to know. Even today, the knowledge still causes me pain, but I have learned to trust in a greater hand than my own because of the error. It is my hope that by disclosing this error others will be able to disclose their mistakes, feel the pain, weep, and then forgive. By including the error, I wept once again as I wrote about it. I touched my sorrow, and then I gained tremendous compassion for myself as a human being.

12/28/99

A month has gone by since I have last written in my journal. Cj returned to the hospital December 24th due to an infection. She went on Mondays, Wednesdays and Fridays for an antibiotic drip (infusion) that lasts about four hours. We thought she was going in on Christmas Eve for the antibiotic but it turned out to be an admission. We were all "bummed" out. Chuck even broke down crying on the phone when he called me. Chuck, Elise and I all cried from disappointment. All Cj had wanted was to be home for Christmas. However, she did get a pass for Christmas Eve and Christmas. I learned how it feels to have a child in the hospital over Christmas. I would not have experienced this otherwise.

Cj has had a wisdom tooth coming in for weeks. It caused her great pain. She slept with me when Chuck went on a business trip to Florida. She slept with both of us for two nights before returning to her own bed. Then on her final night (Thursday) she said she felt safer between us. At least the admission on Friday began her healing. However, Saturday we learned that the G-CFS shots (the shots used to re-start the bone marrow's ability to create blood-producing cells) had to be refrigerated. Cj only trusted me to give her the shots. I learned to give her shots by practicing on an orange. I learned to use a special cream that numbed Cj's skin prior to the shots. But now, we found out that the serum was useless after 24 hours if not refrigerated. I was responsible for giving Cj her shots at home, and I have given her 32 useless shots. Cj only trusted me to give her the shots, but I had not read the small pink print on the box that said to keep these $120.00 shots refrigerated. I missed the small print. Now I realize that it had been insinuated all along that they needed to be refrigerated, but I missed that part. I don't know how; I just did not know.

I experienced one of the greatest errors of my life. I know there are no coincidences — at least for me. I trust that, for some reason, Cj's blood counts were not supposed to come up yet. However, I experienced failure and embarrassment — yet I survived. I survived. I shared this error with others at the time that it happened knowing many would learn from my experience. I even said, "Experience is what you get when you do not read the fine print."

I feel that I am in such turmoil. However, I find I am now trying to touch a feeling rather than analyzing it all the time. So far, it is like touching a butterfly — in attempting to touch it, it lightly flutters away. If I did not try to touch it, it would rest there with its wings closed, and I would not see its beautiful colors. Every time I focused on an uncomfortable feeling my burden lightened, and I realized it floated away. My emotions and physical discomfort were not really so bad.

It is the physiological response that often hurts — this tightness in my chest, in my heart or ache behind my eyes. Stopping the response stifles the feeling. Stifling the feeling only seems to postpone another painful physiological response. Touching the feeling lightens my pain. As I learn to be quiet I will be more in tune to my intuition. I will sense feelings more quickly. I will respond with the intention of universal good rather than co-dependent problem solving.

Eight

Happy New Year

I sat down Monday morning following New Year's Eve and wrote this e-mail to friends. I wrote very little in December. I had been preoccupied with taking care of Cj and doing some things as a family once again. I was continuing to give her the daily G-CFS shots hoping to start the production of blood cells. Cj's Broviac had to be flushed using a very sterile and specific procedure involving four syringes with plastic needles. Cj even learned to do this herself. Cj was going to the hospital as an outpatient three times a week for a four-hour procedure to have an antibiotic infused (slowly dripped into her Broviac) to help prevent infection. While Cj was home we told her we would take her anywhere she wanted to go; we went on a trip to the San Francisco Zoo. Cj said she was more comfortable than anyone on that foggy day because she was in a wheelchair and bundled up in warm clothes.

I continued to work everyday at my job in order to save my sick leave for the time after the bone marrow transplant. I decorated the house for the holidays. I bought and wrapped Christmas presents and put them under the tree. Christmas was Cj's favorite holiday. Cj had been disappointed when we decided not to have our annual Halloween party. I explained that the party was not feasible with her in the hospital. Cj felt better when I promised to decorate the house for Christmas (including the three artificial trees). Then our world again plummeted when Cj had to return to the hospital on Christmas Eve. I did not write until Cj had been back in the hospital for about a week.

01/03/00

Happy New Year and Happy 2000!

Cj saw the year change to 2000 from the 10th floor in the hospital from a window facing San Francisco. Her holidays did not go as she had hoped, but we found a "silver lining" in each experience.

She had stayed out of the hospital for five weeks, up until December 24. The nursing staff made plans for Cj to go for outpatient infusion in the morning on Christmas Eve, so she could make our traditional Christmas Eve dinner at her godparents' home on "Christmas Tree Lane" in Alameda. Blood was waiting to be transfused and the antibiotic waiting for her infusion. Chuck took her to her appointment as I continued Christmas preparations. Cj had insisted that holiday traditions continue. So, one side of the family was coming for Christmas breakfast and the other for a supper buffet.

Chuck took Cj to her appointment at 8:00 a.m. He called at 9:30 a.m. to say that Cj had been admitted to the hospital due to a sinus infection. She would not be coming home. I thought, "All best laid plans go to naught." All Cj wanted was to be home for Christmas. It was a hard blow. We knew Cj had been suffering from pain for four weeks from an emerging wisdom tooth (poor timing), and then we discovered she had a sinus infection.

Cj asked the doctors if she could have a pass for Christmas Eve. They agreed to a three-hour pass if her temperature returned to normal. She received the pass, but not before a family came by and gave her a present. Their son had been in the hospital two years ago on Christmas Eve, and they have returned each year since. Cj also received a gift from the Oakland Police Department. We talked about starting a special Christmas Eve tradition of our own on the way to Alameda next year when Cj is better. We realized that if Cj had come home, we would never have known what it was like to spend a special holiday in the hospital. We would have suspected, but never known.

Cj's temperature went down, and she was also allowed an eight-hour pass for Christmas day. However, she spent most of the day in discomfort. The codeine did not really help her sinus pain, and we forgot to ask for some for home. She felt well enough to open gifts from Santa and our families but not from us. Cj's head hurt, and she asked to go back to the hospital around 6:30 p.m. However, she said she wanted all of our gifts to be taken there. I said she could have a pass on Sunday, and we could celebrate Christmas then. She said, "No." My family loaded up three bags of presents and put them in the car, and the four of us went back to the hospital. After Cj received her pain medication, Chuck, Elise, Cj and I celebrated our Christmas in the hospital room. There were also some anonymous gifts for Cj from the nursing staff. The blessing that we received from this experience is the understanding that Christmas is where our family is.

We made preparations to celebrate New Year's Eve in Cj's room with hats, confetti, noisemakers, sparkling cider and treats. At around 7:00 p.m. a doctor told us an ENT doctor was available to do a procedure to drain and take cultures from Cj's sinuses. Due to a recent blood transfusion, Cj's platelets were up to 60 (meaning her blood could clot), but there was a "window of only six hours" before the platelet count would go back down. Otherwise she would have to wait several days for the procedure. Cultures were needed from her sinus cavities to identify the type infection, determine the best antibiotic and provide the medication necessary to give Cj relief from her sinus pain. Cj said she did not want to miss the New Year's Eve celebration. The ENT doctor said the procedure would take about an hour under conscious sedation, and Cj would be awake before midnight. We knew we did not really have a choice and realized another very important celebration would not go as planned. It was a difficult procedure, and unfortunately, Cj woke up. However, she received a drug that softened her memory of the invasive procedure.

Afterwards, the doctors were amazed that Cj was awake in her room despite taking the maximum adult dose of morphine. I guess Cj was determined not to miss New Year's Eve. She did sleep for a couple of hours after we promised her that we would wake her up before midnight. We awakened her at 11:30 p.m. She mentioned very little about the procedure and had very wide pupils. She said she was "in reality, but the line had become a little less clear." We counted down to midnight and then watched the beautiful fireworks over in San Francisco from Cj's window. Seeing the brilliant colors light the sky above the San Francisco Bay was much more powerful in comparison to seeing them close up on Cj's TV. If we had been home, we would only have watched TV and not known the difference. Also, we would not have experienced the nurses' dedication to making the evening special for all of us.

I am hoping that Cj's sinuses will clear soon. I am anticipating that her white blood count will begin to rise. I look forward to her coming home for a couple of weeks and going out and doing things while she has an immune system. This morning I looked out at the beautiful day thinking it would be nice just to go out for a walk with Chuck. It will come soon enough, and I will look at each step differently.

Nine

Sweet Dreams

I wrote this entry on Saturday while watching Cj, sedated and sleeping, as she was hooked up to tubes and on a breathing machine (ventilator). I did not go to the hospital until later that morning. Cj was awake and alert when I left her around 11:00 p.m. the night before. Chuck usually went earlier to visit with Cj on Saturdays; I usually went in mid-morning and stayed until late at night. Chuck was with her before she went onto the ventilator. One of the most difficult thoughts that I continue to deal with even today is the fact that I never said goodbye to Cj. In my heart I know that father and daughter were to have that final time alone together. However, part of me will always wish that I had gone in early that Saturday, been able to look into her blue eyes one last time and say, "Sweet dreams."

1/15/00

There have been major changes since Monday. Cj is now in ICU at Children's Hospital. She came here late Thursday night after complications from sinus surgery. Chuck and I had a frightening experience in the recovery room when Cj began to choke on blood clots. I yelled several times that she was choking. That got everyone's attention but also got Chuck and I pushed out of the room. I heard "trache" and imagined a tube being put through a hole in the neck. I began to sob and cry.

Everything turned out to be okay. The doctor said Cj had had a spasm in her throat. I felt a great relief. Chuck and I followed her up to her room at Kaiser Oakland. As soon as we got there, she began choking again. Cj's primary nurse, Charlene, pulled out a long narrow clot that looked like a foot-long snake. Then Cj and Charlene pulled out more clots. The doctor decided to send Cj to ICU at Children's Hospital for one-to-one nursing. I stayed with Cj until 1:00 a.m. Interestingly, the clots stopped as soon as she arrived at Children's at 11:45 p.m.

Chuck and I spent Friday helping Cj on and off of the commode. She began having stomach pains early Thursday morning and was unable to do her own toileting care. She had x-rays and scans of her stomach on Thursday, and it is possible that she has typhlitis (an inflammation of the bowel), which can be very dangerous when there is no immune system.

On Saturday morning, Cj sat on the commode while many doctors came in and out of her room. She did refuse to get off and get wiped in front of them. What a difference from the fourteen year-old girl four months ago who locked the bathroom door when she took a bath and initially had to have a blanket held up around her when she first began using the commode.

Cj also has pneumonia. The doctors decided that due to her labored breathing she needed to be put on a ventilator to rest her lungs. When I walked in on Saturday, she was sedated and breathing peacefully and with ease. Chuck told me that the doctors said he could stay with Cj during the procedure. However, Cj looked at him and said, "Dad, you better step out. I don't think you can handle this." I have continued to talk to her as if she is awake and, at times, the machine's beepers go off. The nurse said, "She can hear you."

Cj's body is being taken care of while she is sleeping. She seems to be hooked up to everything: A ventilator, an I.V. for measuring arterial gases, fluids going into her Broviac, and a pulse and oxygen monitor. She is wearing electronic stockings that create alternating leg pressure. I have watched her being turned, changed, cleaned and her lungs suctioned. Her menstrual cycle will not stop, and she has had constant bleeding for weeks. Gynecologists from all over the Bay Area are trying to stop her period but are unsuccessful. It seems that she is making the doctors work very hard for their money.

Later this afternoon, the nurses put in a catheter and diapered Cj. When I walked back into the room she looked like a baby sleeping on her back. She is almost bald with fuzzy hair, diapered and has full cheeks. I wished I could take her into my arms and rock her. Part of me no longer knew what to do. Driving home tonight I thought, "I don't know what I don't know until I know the question." Maybe I need more help asking the questions rather than looking for the answers.

Ten

Taking a Break

This e-mail went to family and friends on a Sunday morning. I wrote it differently from a journal entry since it is a letter rather than an informal entry. I am including this e-mail fully intact, so there are sections that repeat the same information that is in Chapter 9. However, the facts are presented with greater light-heartedness for the sake of our family and friends. There is also information in this letter that was not included in the journal entry. I realized that as I touched the same story over and over again, I recalled more painful details. As I touched different pains, I began to have deeper insights.

1/16/01

Cj Bohntinsky is taking a break. However, her approach has been pretty stressful on Chuck and me. Right now, she is sleeping comfortably. On Thursday, January 13, Cj underwent a CT scan for abdominal pain, a chest x-ray for suspected pneumonia and then went under general anesthesia for surgery on her sinuses. The ENT doctor said the surgery went well, and he led us to the recovery room to be with Cj. She suddenly choked on a blood clot, and I shouted, "She's choking!" That got the attention of everyone as well as getting Chuck and me kicked out of the recovery room. Several nurses came out later (really soon to be honest) and said everything was okay.

About a half-hour later, Cj seemed stable enough to be taken to her room. However, as soon as Chuck, Cj and I reached her room, she began choking again. Chuck and I were pretty devastated and slumped onto the floor outside in the hallway. The staff rushed in, and Cj's nurse, Charlene, removed a large blood clot from her throat. Again, we were told everything was under control, so we went in. There, Cj and Charlene were digging clots out of Cj's mouth as she hacked them up. The clots were large, and you need not know more other than Chuck left.

Charlene made the decision that Cj needed to go to an Intensive Care Unit, which meant a transfer to Children's Hospital in Oakland. She took a clot that she had named "Leroy" down the hall to the doctor. Then I heard her telling the doctor that he'd better guarantee that Cj would receive one-to-one nursing that night. That was not possible on the Kaiser ward so it was off to Children's. I stayed at ICU until 1:00 a.m. and noticed that there were no more clots.

On Friday morning, Cj was continuing to have abdominal pain and beginning to have labored breathing. However, at least there had been no bleeding from her throat since Thursday night. The doctors said they would need to do a bronchoscopy to determine what kind of infection was in Cj's lungs. This meant that a tube had to be put down Cj's throat and into her lungs. The procedure had to be postponed until Saturday due to Cj's risk for bleeding. By Saturday morning, Cj had barely slept for three days. The doctors decided to give her a break. She is now sedated, intubated (a tube down into her lungs) and on a ventilator (breathing machine) in order to give her lungs a rest. Before the procedure, Cj and Chuck kicked the anesthesiologist and doctor out of her room because Cj had to get off the commode. When they returned Cj asked the anesthesiologist, "What are the risks of this procedure? What are the benefits? What are the risks for bleeding?" She was satisfied with the answers so agreed to go to sleep. The doctors told Chuck that he could stay, but Cj said, "Dad, I think you better go out. This is going to be too hard for you to watch." Chuck stayed until she closed her eyes from the gas, and he returned when she was on the ventilator.

Cj is sleeping peacefully. She is once again being well taken care of by a dedicated staff. However, this time her whole body is being taken care of. When I look at her she looks like a baby with her bald fuzzy hair, adult diapers, and plump cheeks. Today I thought it would be wonderful if this was the beginning of the rebirth of her body.

We see Children's Hospital as a new opportunity for us to grow. Everyone here is either a parent, child, or employee. In the cafeteria, we saw parents with ill and injured children. Some were in wheelchairs, some with braces, and one with a raw burned neck. One little girl had scars from burns covering half her face and her right arm, and her left hand was missing. These children are all living; they are all being. They are being themselves and being the greatest teachers that we adults can hope to have. Through our sorrow we can find strength. If the lesson is to disassociate ourselves from our body and to become who we are in the absence of the "perfect" body — then these children are our teachers. If the lesson is that each time we allow ourselves to feel we allow ourselves to heal — then these children are our teachers.

A child died in ICU today. Many had the opportunity to feel sorrow and therefore to heal. Thank you to the children.

Eleven

Who Is to Worry?

I wrote in my journal after a young nurse from Kaiser came by to visit Cj in ICU. She talked gently to Cj as she slept. The nurse smiled at me when she left, but made a guarded comment to Chuck when they happened to meet in the hallway. Chuck was nervous and worried when he entered Cj's room. I realized that I became the most upset when the professional staff shared their worries with us. I had learned that there are no benefits from worrying about the things we can't change or the things we can change. I usually tried not to worry but to do what needed to be done at the time even though it might hurt. However, there were times that I did worry. When I worried, my journal became my best friend. I was beginning to worry so I journaled.

1/17/00

Cj was put on a more powerful ventilator to ease her breathing even more. A special rocking bed was ordered for her because she has pneumonia. The bed will rock her body from side to side to help keep fluid from building up in her lungs.

A Kaiser nurse came by for a visit this afternoon. She seems to be the quiet, concerned, and serious type. I discovered that after she left she bumped into Chuck in the hallway. He told me that she said, "Cj is not out of the woods yet." Now, Chuck was even more worried. He had expressed a lot of worry last night, and I tried to lighten his anxiety. I think the nurse's words undid all I had accomplished last night and earlier today to ease Chuck's anxiety.

I saw Dr. Michaelson when I came in last Saturday. We chatted about the uniqueness and special qualities of children who are seriously ill. He said it was his job to reassure the families and give them hope and for him to take on the worry. I realized that that was why I felt better around Dr. Michaelson than some other doctors. One doctor drained my energy last Friday with his words of concern and his recommendation that we begin praying. I felt a stabbing fear and I paced around Cj's room anxiously for thirty minutes. Fortunately she was sleeping. That doctor released his worry onto me. The nurse did the same to Chuck; she released her worry onto him.

How do I keep my energy high when someone dumps their worries on me? I need my energy to do what is necessary to support Cj and my family. I recognize my energy (or essence within). If it is low or negative due to a worrisome thought, I know I can cancel it. I can cancel my negative thought just as if I pushed delete on the keyboard of a computer. When I say, "Cancel, cancel, cancel," my mind actually registers it as a command to delete that previous thought. I know that this is a powerful tool for lifting up my spirits. I imagine that the worry is rising off my shoulders like a butterfly fluttering away.

Twelve

She Is Still Here

On Tuesday, Chuck and I received pessimistic news from Cj's medical team about her potential for survival. However, her doctors have not give up hope and want to try a special procedure to stop the uterine bleeding. Cj went on a full-power ventilator, and a fungus was found in her sinus cavities. It will probably go to her lungs. She is still on a strange rocking bed to help her lungs.

I went to work Wednesday morning imagining that Cj would be a little stronger when I arrived at the hospital around noon. My plan to stay the morning at work soon changed. I wrote this before leaving my office.

1/19

Last night, I cried the whole time I was with Cj. My tears would not go away. I tried to touch the spot of pain and sorrow, but the butterfly would not flutter away. I would feel peaceful for a moment, but I soon began crying again. I told the ICU nurse that I had been too busy to really weep. It seemed like I had been unable to find a place to weep. I never felt that I could cry in front of Cj because I had to be strong. Last night, I just let myself cry. I touched her face and wept.

When I went into work this morning, I talked to a colleague who is gifted in psychic abilities. She told me several things about Cj. She sensed that Cj was sitting above her bed with her arms crossed and legs folded. (Cj had often sat like that for years.) She said that Cj was tired of being in pain. She wanted her special doll, her room decorated and she wanted her mom. Then this insightful person came back and gave me a note that read, "Touch her and hold her. Read her a story about magic." I knew that meant the Harry Potter book.

I think Chuck, Elise and I are mourning Cj's passing already, although I have not given up hope. The physical things associated with her (her room, toys, books, clothes, etc.) make me break down and weep. I feel better when I think of her essence, that part of her that exists beyond the physical world.

I know we miss Cj. I miss her. I don't know if I am feeling fear of her death. Maybe I am being prepared slowly as her body slowly shuts down. I just miss her. However, I realize that Cj is still here. She has not left yet. I must go home and get her doll. The doll brings such joy to people because it looks and feels like a newborn baby. The nurses played jokes on each other with that doll at Kaiser. I also need to get the book and some of her room decorations. I must go because Cj still needs me; she needs her mom.

Thirteen

There Is Always Laughter

Thursday was our last day with Cj. I wrote this entry in my journal while listening to Chuck read the Harry Potter book to her. His voice shook when he began reading where he had left off a little more than a week ago at Kaiser. "I don't know if I can do this," he said. I assured him that Cj wanted him to read to her. "She can hear you," I whispered.

1/20/00

Chuck, Elise and I are here with Cj. Elise brought Cj's favorite stuffed animal, a dog that she bought Cj when she first became ill. Today is the first time Elise has seen Cj at Children's Hospital. Cj told us that she did not want Elise to visit until she got better. We also brought more things for her room, including Valentine decorations. Pat, the activity director from Kaiser, came by to visit Cj. I mentioned to Pat that I was not sure whether it was legal to put up decorations in an isolation ICU room. I will never forget what Pat told me. She smiled and said, "I believe in asking for forgiveness rather than permission."

At first, it was so hard when I walked into Cj's room this morning and saw her so swollen. She did not look like she was getting better. I felt very hopeless and useless. I thought,

"Where is my miracle? God, you showed me so many miracles over the past four months. I am her bone marrow donor. Where is the miracle of Cj being okay, of her healing?" A gentle voice within responded, "Are you sure you know what the miracle is, or do you have it backwards? Is it her staying or is it her going home?" My soul soared with understanding; my heart sank with sorrow. Then I began stroking her arms and telling her I loved her. I kissed her, touched her, talked to her and tried to listen. Now, I just feel such pain. I am fearful.

Everyone loved Cj's doll. It brought so many smiles to people's faces. It fooled the nurses, doctors and x-ray technician. Charlene, Cj's nurse from Kaiser, visited today and told me that a doctor yelled at her the night before because she was standing beside Cj holding the doll. The doctor wanted to know what she was doing with an infant in an isolation room. The doctor did not believe Charlene when she said it was a doll, so she gave it to him to hold. He was shocked to discover it was not real. Then he smiled and suggested that it would be a great trick on the staff if they took the doll down to the neonatal ward. Charlene smiled, but said the doll was to remain with Cj. Today an x-ray technician came in to x-ray Cj's uterus in preparation for a special procedure. The ICU nurse took the doll from Cj's arm, gave it to me and said, "Here, Grandma." I took the doll and rocked it in my arms. When the technician finished, I said, "Let's give Cj back her doll." The technician's eyes widened. She was amazed that the doll was not real. She told us she thought it was Cj's baby and I was the grandmother. We all laughed. I know Cj was also laughing. Cj was still getting people to find humor even when things were at their worst. Maybe I am learning that laughter does not have to be separate from sorrow. Today is one of the worst days of my life, and there was still laughter.

Fourteen

The Passing . . . A New Beginning

One of the hardest things Chuck and I have ever done was to inform others that we had lost our child. We lost Cj. Cj passed away on Thursday, January 20th. We called family members and let our employers know, but I expressed our loss best through my fingers by typing an e-mail. Family surrounded us for two days. My family — parents, sisters and brother-in laws — came with food and stayed all day Friday. Chuck's mother, stepfather, sister and many cousins came with food and stayed all day Saturday. I wrote this e-mail Saturday morning before Chuck's family arrived. We set up a small memorial altar that included pictures of Cj, her special treasures, her poetry, candles and this e-mail.

1/22/00

We witnessed the most beautiful thing Thursday night on January 20. Cj passed over peacefully and joyfully at 8:35 p.m. with the assistance of an energy healer named Linda. An energy healer is a person trained in cleansing and balancing the electromagnetic body (or aura). When the physical and electromagnetic bodies are in balance one can pass more easily through the tunnel of light. Because of Linda's help, we witnessed a miracle. Cj passed through the tunnel of light at the exact moment of the height of the first lunar eclipse of the millennium. Linda said that is one of the greatest tributes that the universe can give to a soul as it returns home.

Cj never awoke again into the physical world after going onto the ventilator last Saturday. Her lungs worsened, and she became more dependent on the ventilator. No drugs were able to stop her vaginal hemorrhaging. Thursday afternoon the doctors took her downstairs to create a uterine artery embolism to cut off the blood supply to the uterus. As they took her into the room she went into cardiac arrest. Chuck, Elise and I heard the code, "Doctor Hanson STAT to the Catheter Room." We knew that was where Cj was. We thought she was gone at that time. However, a doctor came to us and said that they had quickly revived her, but had decided not to do the procedure. I don't think Cj wanted them to do it, and going into cardiac arrest was the only way she could tell them to stop.

By six o'clock, as we had discussed earlier with the doctors, we stopped all medical intervention except ventilator support and medication for sedation and comfort. I had told Cj on Tuesday that she could go, but I really wanted her to stay. By Thursday afternoon I told her she could go because it was just too hard on all of us for her to try to stay in her body. I knew that Cj could hear us. She knew that we were now ready to handle this loss. Linda was already scheduled to come at 7:30 p.m. I had arranged for her the night before through a colleague at my work. I had originally hoped that Linda was coming to help balance Cj's energy so that her body would begin responding better to the medical treatment. I know now that the Divine Plan had been for Linda to come to help Cj pass over joyfully. The doctors said that Cj would remain on the ventilator and pass away sometime late into the night. I felt it would be so hard just to wait for her last breath, and I asked about stopping the ventilator. The doctors said that it would be best to continue the ventilator, and Cj would slowly slip away as if going into a deep sleep.

That evening, two special friends from my work joined with Chuck, Elise and me, and along with Linda, we formed a healing circle. We spent about ninety minutes touching and caressing Cj. About thirty minutes before her passing, Cj's day nurse came into the room and said, "Cj, thank you for waiting for me." I said, "Luanne, you are off duty." She said she had to come because she'd heard Cj was passing. We all witnessed a miracle of passing. Linda balanced Cj's energy, gave us some messages from Cj and told us where she saw her. At one point, Cj was sitting on a dock at a lake. We did not know of any lake. Then I realized that we had donated some prints to Kaiser's pediatric ward. The nurses loved Cj, and they made sure that a nurse from Kaiser visited her three times a day at Children's Hospital. One print is of two children at a beautiful lake. Cj had gone to visit Kaiser. After awhile, Linda said Cj saw the tunnel of light, and we felt the energy in our bodies intensify as she passed through. Linda said Cj went readily and joyfully. Then Linda moved her hand above Cj's head and chest. I saw Cj's neck muscles moving. Linda did this three times, and each time I saw Cj's neck muscles pulsate. A moment later Luanne said, "Cj is released from her body." I asked how she knew because the monitors were still registering. Luanne said, "Oh, that's just some remaining electrical energy. She has passed over."

A doctor came in and listened to Cj's heart. I heard the doctor ask Luanne, "You've seen many of these. How was this one?" Luanne replied, "This was the most beautiful passing I've ever seen." He then asked if we would like all the tubes removed and then come back in and be with Cj's body. We were grateful. When we went back in, her lavender blanket covered her body, and her head rested on her favorite pillow. She was beautiful. She no longer looked swollen. One devout Catholic colleague looked upon Cj and said she looked like she had transformed into a Buddha. She was beautiful with her soft short fuzzy hair, pudgy cheeks, rounded belly and peaceful expression. The healer said, "Cj is allowing you to see Her." Before passing through the tunnel Linda sensed some messages from Cj. Linda said, "Cj says to lighten up and finish what you start." Cj also said that she will be back because she has so much more to teach! It was hard for us to understand such messages from a child who had just gone through so much suffering.

Elise and Chuck drove home together. I stayed much longer with Cj's body. A nurse from Kaiser came in and offered condolences. My sister, Charlee, did not know that Cj was passing but came by. She sang "Amazing Grace." At the end of the last verse, my pager went off — Chuck had paged me. It was as if Cj were saying, "Mom, call home and go home. This part is over."

I feel joy in her passing. I feel great sorrow and grief in losing her physical body. I feel honored and great joy that Cj chose to come into our family. I feel joy and am humbled to have watched her passing. I feel her around me. I believe that Cj already talks to me. I find great joy in having learned to listen to that gentle Voice within by writing down my thoughts. I never would have dreamed that these lessons were preparing me to be able to listen to the quiet voice of Cj within me. I feel grief in losing her physical body. I feel great joy in having her spirit surrounding us. What is happening in our lives changes moment by moment. God's love never changes, and Cj's spirit will be with us always.

P.S. We are still making arrangements. Cj's body was donated to medical science to help them understand this disease. We will then have her cremated. We will have a memorial service for her, but do not know the specifics yet. They will be revealed in time.

Fifteen

A Special Moment

On Sunday morning, Cj had been gone for three days, and her friends and their parents were coming over. I lay quietly on my back and focused on my breathing. Suddenly, I felt a beautiful and calming energy surrounding me. I felt as if Cj were right beside me, and I thought that if I opened my eyes I might even see her right next to me. However, my sense of her was greater than I had ever felt when she was in her body. I kept my eyes closed and listened to my thoughts. I knew everyone was stunned that Cj passed away. So many of us thought that Cj would get better. I got up and wrote this e-mail and put a copy of it on the altar for everyone to read along with the "The Passing." One parent is a part-time minister. He came up to me after reading "The Passing" and "A Special Moment" and said, "This has changed my life forever."

1/23/00

It has been three days since Cj passed away. I was lying in bed this morning and had a Cj Moment. I felt grief at the loss of her being here with us (in the body). Then I felt the familiar essence of gentle energy surrounding me. She came to me.

Yesterday someone lost a train of thought, and I laughed, saying, "Senior Moment." Last night, Chuck and I were eating dinner alone together, and we thought of Cj. Chuck began to cry, and then I cried, too. "Ah," I said, " a Cj Moment." I realized that we would have many of these moments. I told Chuck that when we suddenly get struck by a thought of Cj and begin to cry, we can just hold up our hand and say, "A Cj Moment."

As I experienced this morning's "Cj Moment," I reflected on her and recalled some memories. Beautiful and funny thoughts came to mind, and I was comforted. I also began to learn and grow. I tried to recall what Cj had taught me during the past few years. One of Cj's statements came to mind: "I believe there is nothing wrong about a lie as long as it does not hurt anyone else." I remember thinking at the time that she had a lot more to learn about life. Now I am not so sure. While talking to a dear physician in the hospital he said, "It is my job to assure and comfort the family and my job to take on the worry." It was when physicians told their direct truth to me that I felt stabs of fear and hopelessness. Once I even had to pace back and forth in Cj's room for about thirty minutes before the fear subsided. I received the worry, and their worries lessened. When I was told, "Others have survived this; do not give up hope," I retained my hope and optimism for Cj's recovery. I remained joyful around Cj. When a loved-one's body is going to cease to exist, I would prefer to have hope and joy up to the very end and then grieve. I watched those who were cautious, very worried and sometimes pessimistic. Their grief is no less than mine is; sometimes I wonder if their grief is even greater.

I wondered about what else Cj had taught me. At first, I could not remember any other statements. Then I recalled a thought I had one day while driving to the hospital: "I do not know what I do not know until I can figure out the question." Cj and I spent many hours together throughout her life because of all her big and little illnesses such as childhood asthma and ingrown toenails. We had many opportunities for conversations that would not have existed otherwise; I would have been at work and she at day care or at school. I realized that she asked me many questions. I do not recall what she asked, but she asked and I answered. I recall Cj once commenting, "Mom, do you know that every time I ask you a question you say you just read about it in a book?" Were her questions reinforcing what I had just learned in a book? During this final illness we spent many hours together at the hospital. When she felt well we had beautiful conversations. She asked me many insightful questions. I answered them the best I could. Each time I gave an answer, I learned a little more. I realized that I was not teaching her spiritual strength, but rather, she was teaching me.

One more thought came to me this morning. "Cj Moments" will always be there for all of us. When we think of her we will have a physiological response of tearing and tightening in the neck and chest. We fear this response. We see it as something negative, and we want to take flight. If we stop for a moment and feel the response, we may find that it is not so scary. Maybe it is Cj saying, "Hi," and asking us to think of her and what she represented. As we get used to this physiological response and no longer fear it, we will learn more from her. She touched each of our hearts differently. She had different messages for each of us. I think Cj would say, "When you feel grief for me knocking, take a deep breath, smile and say, 'A Cj moment.' Smile and think about what I meant to you."

A friend said, "Only if you are happy will Cj be happy in heaven." If you remain sad and unhappy, Cj's life cannot touch you. Feel your body when it says you miss her. Release the fear of grief. Say, "Ah, a Special Moment." Take a deep breath. Smile. Listen to that inner voice within.

Sixteen

What Are My thoughts?

It was a Wednesday morning, and my emotions were fluctuating from a peaceful acceptance of Cj's absence to painful grief.
Part of me kept thinking that maybe this whole thing was a joke
and hoped that Cj would come bouncing through the door any
minute. I always felt so devastated when I thought about how
she was before she got sick. I touched my pain and then sat
down at the computer. I began writing about my thoughts with
a box of tissues nearby.

01/20/01

It is strange how today my body is fluctuating between calm-
ness and that physical stabbing pain that precedes sorrow.
My thoughts really do seem to precede my feelings. What am
I thinking about today?

I had learned over the years that my thoughts actually do af-
fect my being. What is my being? I like to call it my energy. I
am not referring to the energy we often substitute for the
word willpower. I may say I do not have the energy to go out,
or go to work, or exercise, or cook tonight, etc. This is willpower. Either I have the willpower to do something or not.

My true energy, the life force that radiates around and through me, is influenced by my thoughts. At first, I practiced sensing energy changes by smiling and frowning. When I smiled, I felt more uplifted and happier. When I frowned, I actually felt my body and energy slump. Later, I moved into practicing with my thoughts. I learned that judgements caused my energy to slump; acceptance made me feel light and peaceful. Interestingly, and somewhat hard to accept at first, I discovered all judgements gave me a sense of an energy slump. If I said something was good or right versus bad or wrong, I felt the same energy slump. At first this confused me. Then I remembered an ancient saying, "Judge not lest ye be judged." It does not say to make only positive judgements but to "judge not." I realized that all my judgements came right back at me by lowering my energy or life force.

For several years I have focused on the concept of non-judgement. I realized that what I thought was good or right another person may have thought was bad or wrong. Also, each time I judged something I knew my energy lowered, regardless of whether my judgement was positive or negative. Being a rather judgmental person, I felt at a loss regarding what I could think about and still keep my energy high. Then I recalled a powerful recommendation, "It is important to express your feelings." I knew that this recommendation suggests that I use the words, "I feel" rather than "you are." For example, I felt okay if I thought, "I feel sad when you do not talk to me." I felt depleted of energy if I thought, "You are not considerate because you do not talk to me." With the first thought, I am taking responsibility for my feelings. In the second thought, I am blaming my situation and discomfort on someone else.

I learned to try to think in the terms of feelings. My energy stayed high when I thought, "I don't like the way that person acted." I was not judging the person, I was expressing how I felt, including what I liked or did not like. When I thought, "I like what that person said," my energy still stayed high. Little did I know that I would be applying these lessons to dealing with my daughter's illness and death. So, what are my thoughts? I know that my energy will stay high if I express how I feel, what I do or don't like, and do not judge the situation. I know that I will feel pain when I express how I feel, but I also know I will continue to heal as I continue to write this. I think I will cover what I did not like first, as I usually like to save the best for last.

I do not like writing down things I did not like or journaling my worries. I do not like the fact that I had to draw on over twenty years of experience working in a hospital with patients and families devastated by strokes and head injuries and then became "one of the family members." But I am concerned about the statements that we received from the physicians, nurses, and social worker that they had not seen families handle their children's illnesses with such love, compassion and humor previous to Cj. I do not like the fact that other families did not know how to handle tragedy in a less agonizing way. I have appreciated the encouragement to share our experience and "wisdom" with as many people as possible. A great part of my experience was through my thoughts, because it is primarily through my thoughts that I experience the world. It is through my thoughts that I have gained insight into myself. So, what are my thoughts?

I don't like the fact that my daughter got sick. I didn't like hearing her diagnosis and the seriousness of it. I don't like the fact that her illness is rare and her treatment was part of a national study due to the need for research on myelodysplastic syndrome. I didn't like cutting off her curls. I didn't like her being isolated from her friends. I didn't like seeing her hunched over due to discomfort from the surgery for insertion of the Broviac (the small tube close to her heart for receiving medications instead of having to be poked with needles for I.V. lines). I didn't like watching her receive chemotherapy. I didn't like watching her hair fall out and seeing the black roots that she called "singed." I didn't like watching her throw up neon green and have diarrhea.

I didn't like watching her pull one or two I.V. poles holding medication-dispensing machines to the bathroom with her. I didn't like her lack of appetite. I didn't like giving her shots. I didn't like flushing her two Broviac lines (the two tubes that hung outside of her chest) to keep them from clogging. I didn't like knowing that any deviation from this cautious cleansing procedure could cause an infection to go directly to Cj's heart. I didn't like it when I accidentally hurt her by pulling on her Broviac lines. I didn't like it when she yelled at me. I didn't like her lack of exercise. I didn't like fearing that anything she touched could make her ill due to the absence of an immune system. I didn't like her wisdom tooth coming in after her second round of chemotherapy and the pain it caused her. I hated learning about the error regarding storing the G-CFS shots. I didn't like her pain and headaches. I didn't like her going back into the hospital on Christmas Eve. I didn't like her pain from sinusitis. I didn't like her receiving a sinus flushing under conscious sedation on New Year's Eve and knowing that she had awakened during the procedure. I didn't like her drowsiness and reduced awareness due to the morphine. I didn't like her sinus surgery and her spiting up clots of blood. I didn't like her going to the Intensive Care Unit (ICU) at Children's Hospital.

I didn't like seeing her having trouble breathing and not sleeping. I didn't like hearing that she was very sick. I didn't like walking past all the other very sick children in ICU to reach Cj's isolation room. I didn't like seeing her in an induced comatose state on the ventilator with a tube in her mouth for almost a week. I didn't like the fact that I had not been there to say, "I love you," before she went on the ventilator (although her dad was there). I didn't like seeing her in diapers. I didn't like hearing the nurse pleading with the blood bank for more blood and platelets. I didn't like watching Cj receiving so much blood and so many platelets. I didn't like watching her continued uterine bleeding and each time the doctors tried a new drug to stop it, hearing that it did not work.

I didn't like not knowing if she heard me when I talked to her or felt my touch when I embraced her hands and arms or massaged her feet. I didn't like telling her she could go if she wanted. I didn't like thinking she had died down in the procedure room when they were trying to stop the uterine bleeding. I didn't like it when we agreed with the doctors not to do any intervention if her heart stopped again. I didn't like it when we told the doctors to stop all blood transfusions. I didn't like it when she passed away. I didn't like taking down the Valentines and other decorations in her room.

I didn't like balancing going to the hospital and work. I didn't like worrying about taking too much time off from work, thinking I would need my leave time later during Cj's illness. I didn't like worrying about what would happen if I had to take a leave of absence. I didn't like worrying about how I was going to get to San Francisco every day after Cj's bone marrow transplant. I didn't like worrying about what would happen if Cj needed extensive care at home as her immune system recovered. I didn't like worrying about our future.

I've heard that when we give we receive so much more in re-turn. We gave our daughter so that so many more people can learn to embrace the joys that accompany sorrow — if only they have eyes to see and an open heart to feel. What are my joyful thoughts?

I loved spending hours alone with my daughter, talking and listening to music. I loved the beautiful talks we had to-gether. I liked writing about what I had learned from our conversations, including how to cherish each moment of life. I liked seeing Cj's desire to help others even though she was facing a serious life challenge. I loved seeing her smile at oth-ers and listening to her talk to those she liked. I appreciated hearing how much the medical staff enjoyed their time and chats with Cj. I liked hearing the medical staff's amazement at how Cj took responsibility for knowing about her medica-tions and treatment. I liked how she only trusted me to give her the injections. I loved knowing I was her bone marrow match and was often walking right beside her.

I loved decorating Cj's hospital room. I loved taping all her get-well cards to the walls. I loved putting up the decorative flags of the unicorn and the tulips. I enjoyed the twinkling beaded curtain that we attached to her wall. I loved putting photographs and special statuettes on the counters. I loved bringing in her three-dimensional balloons, especially the butterflies. I loved putting up decorations for each holiday — Halloween, Thanksgiving, Christmas and New Year's Eve. I liked how enthused everyone was about her room and how the nurses referred to Cj's room as "the place to be." I loved it when Cj told me her nurses often took their breaks in her room.

I loved watching her do her art projects while in the hospital. She sculpted tiny elves, one sitting on a mushroom and one on a tree stump. One was for the social worker and the other for me. She sculpted a beautiful rose for her sister and a boy fishing for her dad. She learned to do cross-stitch and completed a design of hummingbirds. I love seeing it framed in her bedroom.

I rejoiced at hearing the words, "Cj can go home." I loved having Cj at home. I liked knowing that we were competent to continue with her medical care at home. I enjoyed seeing her friends come over and visit her. I liked seeing her on the couch watching TV. I liked knowing Elise was spending time with her. I liked buying her new pajamas. I liked watching Cj and her friends put up the Dickens villages for the holidays.

I appreciated how the nurses and doctors welcomed Cj as a friend when she returned to the hospital. I liked that she received a pass on Christmas Eve and saw the Christmas lights she had seen every year since an infant. I loved Cj's insistence on continuing our holiday traditions. I was grateful for her pass to come home on Christmas even though she was in pain. I enjoyed our personal family Christmas celebration in the hospital even though I felt a little uncomfortable carrying in three large bags of gifts. I liked seeing gifts waiting for her from the Oakland Police Department. I appreciated the fact that I learned through experience what it was like to have an ill child spend Christmas in the hospital.

I appreciated all the get-well cards that Cj received. I appreciated the little gifts that people brought or sent her. I appreciated it when Cj had visitors, although at times she said she only wanted the immediate family with her. I appreciated words of concern and encouragement from family, friends and co-workers. I liked writing e-mails and letters telling about recent experiences, what they meant to us and what we learned from each. I liked hearing that everyone read the e-mails and letters and that our correspondence not only touched their hearts but also helped them to cope with our pain.

I appreciated the hope that I continued to have for Cj up to the very last hours of her life. I appreciated the doctor who said it was the physician's job to take on the worries and to give the family hope. I appreciated the doctors who continued to give us hope even while being honest with the severity of Cj's illness. I treasured the opportunity to finally mourn the whole experience, crying and holding Cj's hand while she lay unconscious on the ventilator. (There had never been a good time to lament and weep.) I appreciated the doctors' honesty when it was time to let Cj go. I respected our ability and readiness to let her go.

I loved touching her and putting pure lavender oil on her head, face, arms and legs. I loved that Elise and I sprinkled her with "fairy dust" (a fine glittery powder that one of my sisters had sent in a get-well card). I am thankful that we had someone who would help her pass over in the manner of our faith. I am thankful for the select eclectic group of friends who joined us in facilitating Cj's passing. I was amazed at the ICU nurse who suddenly came in to join us on her day off. I appreciated the special doctors who dropped in to say good-bye. I will always remember the young doctor who said, "Cj, you were the bravest of the bravest." After Cj passed, I appreciated the doctor who came in, listened to Cj's heart and asked, "Would you like all the tubes removed and then come back in and spend some time with her?"

I love my final memory of Cj. Her favorite lavender blanket covered her, and her head was on her favorite pillow. Her face was beautiful and full of peace. Much of the swelling in her face had suddenly gone down. She sparkled with fairy dust. I, a person who had a phobia of being near death all my life, found myself in awe over her peace and beauty. I loved holding her hand and touching her face. Even though Chuck and Elise finally went home, I could not leave. I love that my younger sister suddenly showed up. I love that she sang, "Amazing Grace." I then love my memory of being tickled when my pager went off, and it was my home number. I felt it was as if Cj were saying, "Mom, this part is over, it is time to go home." I love that this end is only a new beginning.

Seventeen

The Memorial Preparations

We took our time to plan for the memorial service. It was on Saturday, nine days after Cj passed away. As the pastor said, "There are no precedents when it comes to memorial services." I had wrapped Cj's ashes in beautiful fabric tied with a gold rope. However, the task was not easy, and I hugged her ashes and rocked them back and forth as I wept over our loss. Part of me was so tired of weeping, so tired of the pain. I had never liked funerals or memorial services because they always hurt my heart, and I cried easily. Now I had to face the scariest service of all — my daughter's. I wrote in my journal before going to the service.

1/28/00

We spent yesterday preparing the church fellowship hall for the memorial service. Teal was to be the color for some reason. Chuck, Elise, and I were busy setting up the flags, balloons and beads that had decorated Cj's hospital rooms. We put up a memory board of pictures spanning from her newborn photographs to a picture of her standing bald and smiling next to the Christmas tree in November. Beautiful flowers arrived from Mom and Dad. The pastor worked with us setting up chairs, and Mom and my brother, Fred, helped set the tables. Later, Mom and Dad took all of us out for dinner.

Last night, we also picked up Elise and her friends from the Little Theater after the play, "Rumors" ended. There I bumped into a friend that I had not seen for years. I was so happy I had thought to call her this afternoon to tell her of Cj's passing. It would have been almost impossible to tell her the news while standing outside of the theater and impossible not to tell her.

We arrived home around 11:00 p.m. and Chuck and I started cleaning the kitchen. We began listening to a CD by Andrea Bocelli, and I started crying. I realized that I had been feeling angry. I wept an angry grief. I wept for the world. I wept for the pain that all people go through when they discover a loved one is seriously ill or after a soul has passed. I do not believe that such occurrences are a cruel act of God but are part of the beautiful lessons that we can receive on earth. I find that each time I feel pain, I feel sorrow. Each time I feel sorrow, I weep. Each time I weep, I heal. Each time I heal, I grow. The cycle is pain, sorrow, healing, and growth. Without feeling pain we do not grow; we refuse to change.

I think that many people fear change. Change makes us face the unknown. So often it seems easier and much more comfortable to do the same thing every day: to think the same thoughts and act the same way. Change causes me to expand beyond my standard way of doing or thinking about something. Interestingly, when I think of expanding I think of stretching. When I have stretched my muscles I often feel some pain and then a painful stiffness the following day. When I stretch my mind by studying new concepts I may get a headache. Stretching is an experience that expands my capabilities such as my body's flexibility, my knowledge base or my understanding about life. That stretching seems to cause an initial discomfort. I believe that my greatest growth can come through allowing myself to experience and touch my pain and sorrow from the loss of Cj.

Many years ago, I learned a management concept called the "Valley of Despair," but I never knew I would have to draw upon it during a time of sorrow. When we make a change, things often get worse. Then, over time, things actually are better than before. It looks like a "check mark." The valley of despair is at the bottom of the check mark where things are at their worst. I feel I'm in the valley of despair right now. I feel despair for myself, for my husband, for my daughter, for our families and friends. I do not believe that I can go any lower than this.

I've heard that one has to hit bottom before beginning to heal. I thought this was only for people with addictions. Now I realize it is for many of us. I believe I have hit bottom within the "valley of the shadow of death," and I no longer fear sorrow. The Divine has comforted me throughout Cj's illness, during her passing and after the loss of her presence. Some Divine Force continues to comfort me. My greatest Comfort comes when I ask for it. When I ask to be cradled in God's arms and embraced by the Universe, I feel my pain being eased and a gentle peace surrounding me.

Today I have to go to the memorial service. Chuck says it is not only for our families and friends, but also for me. So I will go. I will watch, listen and speak when moved. I will weep, and then I shall celebrate with a beautiful cake, sweets and music. Today I will again experience pain over the loss of Cj's presence. I will have sorrow, I will weep, I will heal and I will grow.

Thank you, Cj, for choosing me as your mother. Thank you for all the lessons that you taught me. Thank you for the lessons that you continue to teach me. I know the lessons will continue, but they will be gentler. I have been through the "Valley of Despair." I no longer fear sorrow. If I do not fear sorrow then I will not fear the pain of change. I will embrace it and know that it is the way of growth.

Eighteen

The Memorial

The memorial service was over and I wanted to remember the details. So I decided to write down some notes about how it went. However, as I wrote about the service, I began to write about my thoughts and feelings. In returned I received insights and felt another part of myself heal.

1/28/01

Today was the day of Cj's memorial service. We refilled the Mylar balloons that had floated above Cj in her hospital rooms: five butterflies, a snail, a caterpillar, and a ladybug. Then Chuck and I picked up the beautiful lavender and purple sheet cake. Several of Elise's friends were already at the church, and they helped us bring things into the fellowship hall. I was so surprised by all the beautiful flower arrangements that filled the room. We had requested donations to the CJ Foundation in lieu of flowers. Suddenly, I realized how beautiful the flowers were and how they brought life to the room.

We arranged a table that displayed pictures of Cj, her poems, and a prized certificate she had received in third grade. She had kept the certificate on her wall for over five years. She had received an outstanding achievement award for weaving a beautiful tapestry and conducting an amazing puppet show. I shook my head and reflected on life every time I looked at that certificate. We received several sympathy cards that had talked about how we would understand the tapestry of loss when we viewed it from the other side.

The table also displayed my father's Purple Heart from World War II. He gave his medal to Cj in November for her valor in fighting her illness. She loved the medal and showed it to the doctors and the nurses. My father designed a certificate to go with it that read:

"For courage and determination above and beyond
that demanded of most individuals,
Cj Bohntinsky,
despite illness, adversity, pain, discomfort
and change in personal appearance,
has constantly displayed
an interest and concern for others,
both adults and children, that has brightened their lives,
maintained their spirits and allowed them to carry on in
their daily activities and anxieties,
is awarded the Purple Heart
by Granddad Fraser,
recipient in 1945 for being run over by a tank."

I went into the kitchen and arranged a bouquet of tropical flowers sent to us from a friend in Hawaii. I kept thinking about the color teal and what it meant. I had felt the need to buy teal tablecloths and tableware. Later, I noticed that the color of the parish hall was teal. I reflected on what teal might represent. Suddenly an idea came to me. The color was not teal; the color was aqua. I thought that aqua might represent the Age of Aquarius. I realized that there must have been something about Cj choosing Hawaii for a family vacation and both she and Elise meeting my old friend Michael. I wondered if something about Cj represented the beginning of the Age of Aquarius. Did Cj represent a new way of healing from sorrow?

The service started with a lament on the bagpipes. Cj wanted to learn to play the bagpipes and march in a band, and we had found an instructor for her just about the time she became ill. Then, Chuck stood up to speak about Cj. He talked about Cj's birth and how he always suspected that she had winked at him when he took her from the doctor's arms. I do not remember anything else he said, but I do remember feeling that Chuck would be okay. Then he read the poem Cj wrote about herself in September. One line of Cj's poem said that she would like to see the end of world hunger. While listening to Chuck read her poem, I realized that Cj was not just talking about food. She was talking about world hunger for peace and understanding, for the release from fear of suffering, for the comfort that God gives when we ask for it, for the ability to be comforted, and world hunger for trusting in the Universal design of the Great Tapestry.

Friends and family took turns telling stories about Cj. She loved to tell and listen to stories. One friend recalled Cj helping her at a tea party and carrying very heavy pots without any complaints. Chuck's boss talked about our Halloween parties and how Cj took her son's hand (when he was four) and gently led him through the hallways of goblins, devils and witches so he could be with the big kids upstairs. My father stood, using his two canes for support, and described Cj's determination in painting their one-rail fence that circled the front yard. No one knew that Cj was sick when she was painting the fence. Others told about the impact Cj had on their lives.

Many came to the service, and we greeted people we had not seen for years. Cj's main doctor, Dr. Month, and the nurses from both Kaiser and Children's Hospitals came. Elementary school teachers and the principal came. Middle school and high school teachers came. People from my work and Chuck's work came. Our parents' friends came. Our friends came. Godparents came and Cj's and Elise's daycare parents came. Many people came to honor Cj, to comfort us and to be comforted.

When the service ended, we celebrated with Cj's favorite food — sweets, including the sheet cake and cookies. Later, we heard that people stood by the cake and stared at it before taking any pieces. The words on the cake were Cj's comments that came through when she passed away. The cake read, "Cj says, 'Lighten up. Finish what you start. I came to teach.' " I later asked why people were staring at the cake. I discovered that beautiful celebration cakes were rarely at memorial services. People loved the cake.

Later, we received feedback that the memorial service surprised many people. They had expected a funeral-type service. We held the entire service in the church's reception hall in order to make people of all faiths feel comfortable. There were many children and teenagers; some had never been in a church. We had decided that we wanted the service to be a celebration of Cj's life and her passing, while also recognizing our pain and sorrow in losing her. It was a healing experience. A group of teenagers played in a band afterwards and entertained people with fun music. Later that night, we counted over 250 signatures in the guest book. We were told that everyone did not sign the guest book because the service had already been delayed over 20 minutes due to people signing the book.

I felt blessed that our whole family received Divine strength to make it through the memorial service without breaking down. Chuck and I had wept the night before. We mourned and grieved over Cj's absence. I told myself and others that we had cried a lot the night before so maybe the Divine was being merciful with us. We were able to comfort others and accept their comfort so much better by not weeping on this day. We had touched our sorrow the night before and God was merciful today. Chuck was right — part of the memorial service was for me. It is a day I will always remember and cherish.

Nineteen

Thank You, Doctor

We received a heart-felt letter from an anesthesiologist at Children's Hospital about a week after Cj passed away. His words touched our hearts and helped give meaning to Cj's illness and death. Since he took the time to write a two-page letter by hand, I felt moved to send him a thank-you note. I knew that people often needed to share information about a tragedy many times to help heal the wounds. Writing this thank-you letter gave me an additional opportunity to express our loss, to touch my pain and heal a little more.

January 30, 2000

Dear Dr. Rowe,

Thank you so much for your beautiful and heartfelt letter regarding Cj's illness. Your letter provided us additional inspiration to make Cj's passing meaningful. We feel so humbled each time we find that Cj's illness and passing made a difference in someone's life. Although we received a nice card from the Grievance Committee, it was not helpful in healing our grief. Your letter was a beautiful gift that helped us heal.

Cj's illness and passing will continue to benefit many. Over the next couple of months we will establish the CJ Foundation. Its purpose will be to help lessen the anguish that family member's experience when a child is diagnosed with a life threatening illness. This will be accomplished through education and charitable giving. I've had many talks with Kim, the social worker at Oakland Kaiser. Kim told us she had never seen a family handle an illness the way we handled Cj's. At first, we thought everyone handled illnesses the way we did. We had never been through a life-threatening illness before, especially with a child. However, we discovered, and were assured, that we had something to share to others. Your letter gave us additional motivation to take on the task of writing a book and creating a foundation.

I am blessed to have worked in a medical center for over 20 years. I am a speech pathologist and have worked in the rehabilitation of adults in acute medical, acute rehabilitation, neurorespiratory, and skilled nursing throughout my career. I never dreamed that I would have to apply my knowledge, skills and compassion to my daughter. Soon after Cj's illness was diagnosed on September 17, 1999, I shared with my family that we would write a book on the experience. It is called *The Healing Room.* Throughout her illness, Chuck and I kept journals of her situation, including our feelings, sorrows, and what we were learning from each experience. I kept looking for the healing room. I thought it was in the first hospital room, then at home, then back at the hospital, then in ICU, then in the conference room when we were deciding to let Cj go, then at home and finally at the memorial service. I now realize the healing room is in the heart.

I wrote many e-mail letters to our family, friends and co-workers to keep them up-to-date on Cj's illness. I talked about her reactions to chemotherapy in the hospital and at home. We shared our Christmas celebration at home (Cj had a pass) and in the hospital. We wrote about celebrating New

Year's Eve at the hospital, Cj's transfer to ICU at Children's Hospital and her beautiful passing at Children's. Thank you so much for your help in making that possible. We shared what each experience meant to us and what we learned. We received feedback that these letters were helping others deal with Cj's illness. We were asked if we were saving the e-mails. We soon realized that these e-mails and journal entries were all part of the book. We were writing the book all along.

Cj once told me that one of her greatest fears was of being disappointed. I told her that I believed that the feeling of disappointment would be just as strong whether you looked forward to the event or worried that the event would not happen. Throughout Cj's illness she saw people who did not give up hope for her recovery; not her family, not her friends and not the medical field. However, there were some people who were pessimistic. I discovered that the sorrow and grief was just as strong for those who had been cautious as for those who hoped and had faith. In fact, I wonder if the cautious ones experienced even more grief.

I am enclosing copies of some of the e-mails we sent to our friends. One friend said he sent them to another friend who was facing a family member's life threatening illness. Thank you for your prayers. Embrace your daughters; they are the lights of the world.

Twenty

The "Might Have Beens"

A few days following the memorial service, Chuck and I began driving past places that Cj had frequented. We cried as we drove past her middle school. I realized that these were "Cj Firsts" and understood that pain would hit and tears would flow the first time we did something that reminded us of Cj. We cried during our first dinner as a family of three, but the second dinner was easier.

In early February, Chuck and I drove up to his parents' home in the mountains. It was the first time that we had driven up there without any children. Cj was gone, and Elise was in school. About half way to his parents, I began to feel that stabbing pain in my chest. I wiped tears from my eyes. I pulled out my journal and wrote.

020400

Driving up to Cj's grandparents' house in the mountains has brought that tight pain to my chest and the familiar tears as soon as I realized that this was our first trip to the mountains alone. Elise is in school. Chuck and I realized that in the future we would only go up to the mountains as a family of three or just as the two of us.

The Healing Room

I remembered the place that is about halfway to Chuck's parents' where they met us and took Elise and Cj to their home for a few days. We'd meet at a burger place, chat and then watch them all drive off together. Later, we met again at the burger place to pick up the girls and listen about their trip. We both cried when we passed that meeting place. We knew it was another "Cj First." How many Cj Firsts are in store for us? I do not know.

While riding in the car, I began reflecting on the Cj Firsts and realized my pain came from experiences that triggered memories of the past. Chuck or I would feel pain, cry, and then one of us generally said, "I miss Cj." I reflected on that statement. What did we miss? I had my memories just like when she was with us. Chuck and I always talked about the kids, joyfully reliving memories. The stories of Cj's mischief always made everyone laugh. These stories are still with us. The memories did not pass. Therefore, with Cj's passing we did not lose the memories and stories.

I say that I miss Cj's presence. In thinking back, I realized she was often away from us over the past several years. She was busy with school, homework, friends, watching TV, working on the computer, hammering things outside or playing alone in her room. Often over dinner, I'd say, "This is the only time we really have together because you kids are off doing your own thing." Sometimes I felt like I saw them fifteen minutes a day. If this is true, why do I feel such pain at missing her presence?

Is it really her body, her smile, her voice that I miss? I think one thing I really miss right now is the "What Might Have Beens." As a parent, I had so many dreams for Cj. She wanted to be a kindergarten teacher. She loved children and she had such a gift for knowing what each child needed to feel special. I had visions of her as a teacher with the children hugging her waist. I knew she would make a wonderful mother and contribute to the world by raising insightful children. I looked forward to being a grandmother. I looked forward to her family seated around our dinner table.

Cj and I often went together to see movies that neither Chuck nor Elise wanted to see. I looked forward to those special times when she and I would continue to go to movies together when I was old. I looked forward to our shopping trips and even buying things for her children. I looked forward to our talks and trying to figure out what life is all about. I looked forward to learning all that she had to teach me through her questions and later through her answers.

I realized a great part of my pain was the loss of what might have been. I lost my dreams and visions for my fourteen-year-old daughter. I can tell myself that those dreams may never have happened anyway. We never really know the future. However my heart aches at losing those dreams and hopes for what might have been.

Twenty-one

Once Upon a Lunar Eclipse

In the beginning of February, I saw an advertisement in the newspaper inviting amateur poets to submit a poem. I wondered why I had discovered it. I no longer believed in coincidences, but I was not even an amateur poet. I had never written a poem except, "Roses are red," so why was I reading this invitation to enter a poem into a contest? I realized that I never believed I could write until I began to journal. Now, my journal entries were beginning to surprise me. I noticed that my writing had deepened since Cj passed away. Could I possibly write a poem? I decided to try. I wrote this poem in less than half an hour and submitted it. I did not win a prize, but my poem was published in 2000 in a book of poems called *The Lightness of Being*.

I learned that there was more than one way to journal. I could journal in my formal journal book with its pretty cover. I could journal on a piece of scrap paper. I could journal on the computer. Now, I could also journal by writing a poem. I learned even more about myself because I was willing to write a poem.

Once Upon a Lunar Eclipse

Sorrow turned into magic once upon a full lunar eclipse.
Tears turned into smiles as she floated through the light.
Fears turned into trust as we felt a little bit of heaven.

Pain turned into awe as she lay there in lavender;
	her body finally at peace.
Grief turned into thanks for the fourteen years she stayed.
Thanks turned into loneliness for her blue sparkling eyes,
	songs and smiles.
Loneliness turned into anguish over times we'd no longer
	share.
Tears turned into reflections over reasons for her leaving.
Reflections turned into healing; lessening the pain
	from our child's passing.
Healing turned into growth as we discovered
	the purpose for death's visit.
Knowing turned into joy over love never to be forgotten.
Sorrow turned into magic once upon a full lunar eclipse.

In memory of Christen Jean Bohntinsky

Twenty-two

Regrets
(An Essay by Elise)

When Elise was a junior in high school and had an assignment to write about a personal experience, she knew immediately what she was going to write about. Elise and I had talked about the importance of touching our pain. She often watched me journal after I cried. I was never quite sure if my ideas were helping her. I cried when Elise shared this essay with me. Elise had touched one of her most painful feelings and she grieved. She even shared her pain, regrets and lessons with her teacher by writing this essay. I felt that once again, Cj's passing was touching others.

020700

"Elise, the doctors don't think that Cj is going to make it."

Those were words that I thought I would never have to hear. Sure I had contemplated the possibility that I wouldn't grow old with my sister, but I never believed that it would actually happen. However, on January 20, around 8:30 p.m., I lost the best friend that I had ever had. After struggling for four months with Myelodysplastic Syndrome, a disease similar to leukemia, Cj got to go home. Not to the home that she had known for 14 years, but to the one that she left when she was born. She was simply too bright of a soul to remain here.

I kept waiting to feel emotions that I believed to be typical after loss: denial, anger, and depression. However, those feelings didn't come. I thought that maybe passing away was the best thing for my sister. Who would want to come back only to experience more pain and suffering? I was filled with only one feeling, regret; regret that I hadn't spent more time with her.

I had always believed that Cj was unique. She was outgoing, made friends with everyone easily, and livened up any room that she entered. Cj was never afraid to say what she thought, regardless of consequences. She wore what she wanted which usually meant many clashing colors and patterns; she hated to match. She had the confidence that I desired; yet sometimes I was embarrassed to have her with me because of the stares that she received. She lived for those stares, always trying her hardest to get a reaction out of someone. It wasn't until after her death that I realized how special she really was.

Cj had always been one of my best friends. We shared our hopes, dreams, and fears while sitting up late at night talking. I could trust her with any secret and in turn she trusted me. During our conversations we realized that we envied each other. She wanted the close relationships that I had with my friends while I desired the confidence that she displayed to the world. Cj considered me her best friend, but I took our friendship for granted and put others ahead of her. I am angry with myself that I didn't treat her as a true best friend until it was too late. It was September when I really began to spend quality time with her. We listened to music, colored, talked about the past, present, and future, and watched movies that we had always enjoyed.

Everyone told me that we were the closest sisters that they had ever seen. They were amazed at how many places I took her, and how much time I spent with her. Nevertheless, I know that I could have done more. I am ashamed to know that I put my desires ahead of her more times than I care to think about. I wish that I had just stayed to watch movies and talk with her instead of going to a concert with my friends. She always tried her hardest to make me happy. I regret that the same isn't true for me. She was one of the most cheerful and brightest souls that I have ever encountered; being with her would always brighten my day. I was blessed that she was my sister; however, I simply didn't realize how precious my time with her really was.

When Cj got sick I began to realize how much we had been drifting apart. She had commented on it before but I hadn't wanted to believe it. I'm glad that I at least tried to make up for all the disappointment I had caused her over the years. For the last four months we had reclaimed the best friend status, but I still took her for granted. My needs still came first, even when she was home, taking a break from the hospital. Although we did spend time coloring, talking, laughing, and watching movies together, I still spent too much of my free time with my friends.

Instead of seeing my friends, I could have spent the precious days I didn't know were numbered with her. By the time we realized that she might pass away I hadn't seen her in a week. She hadn't wanted me to visit her. She said that it would be too hard on me to see her in so much pain. When I finally went to visit her she was already in an induced comatose state. A tube was doing most of her breathing and she was unable to respond to my voice. I didn't get to hear her voice one last time. I didn't get to cherish every last day I had with her. Now I would give anything for just five minutes to say goodbye and that I love her.

I know that many people share similar feelings. Her friends who only saw or talked to her once or twice during her illness are also experiencing regret. They wish that they could have just one more phone call or just one more visit. We all carry some type of regret with us. Cj has taught us all something very important; to cherish what we do have and those we love, just as she did.

It's simply human nature to put our hopes, dreams, and desires above those of the people around us and then to regret it when someone we love is no longer here. When a painful experience has to teach us that this isn't the way to live life, the lesson sticks with us. I know that from now on I will treasure every moment I have with my friends and family. I will try to make their happiness coincide with my own, not teeter below it.

I am still filled with many regrets that I know will last my lifetime. Comfort is found only when I remind myself that Cj knows that I still love her unconditionally. She understands why I acted the way I did. I hope that my regrets will help me to make better and wiser decisions in the future, even if they sadden me in the present.

Twenty-three

A Letter to Cj

It was a Friday evening, and I ached with grief. I was alone and seemed to be crying constantly. I realized that it had been exactly three weeks since Cj passed away. I had read in a booklet that writing a letter to the loved one who passed away could be helpful during a time of grief. I had not even written Cj a letter when she was living, and I never wrote anyone who had died before. However, my heart ached, so I sat down at the computer and wrote this letter.

021100

Dear Cj,

Oh, how I miss you. I want you to come home. I wish that this was all a big joke and you would walk through the door. I love you so much. My heart aches for you. My tears flow for you. I am so sorry that you got sick and that there was nothing we could do to stop the progression of your illness. We tried everything we could think of. You were so brave throughout the process.

Sometimes I do not feel brave in going through this grief process. I know it is necessary for healing, but it hurts so much. I went back to work this week. I do not like work right now.

The people are caring and understanding, but I get tired of them asking me how I am doing. It is such a natural question. The problem is that I don't think I really know how I am doing. I know my feelings best when I am crying because I am grieving. But how am I doing when I am busy doing the tasks of my job and not feeling sorrow at that immediate moment? I know some people are uncomfortable around someone who has experienced a tragedy, especially the death of their child. These people do not say anything to me at all. So far I like the, "Welcome back. We missed you. Remember, your work family is here for you." Those were the most comforting remarks from a co-worker.

I do not like the stress of work at all. I find myself impatient and resentful. Some people are clueless regarding how to speak to a person experiencing grief, or even how to speak to people in general. How nice it would be to receive a simple, "I know times are difficult, but would it be possible for you to do such and such?" How much nicer than, "Did you get your report in?" I have enough stress just trying to stay focused on my work and not breaking into tears. Maybe it would have been better if I had just looked at the person and started crying instead of saying, "I will get it to you." If tears really do release strain than I would have felt better. Instead I felt anger and resentment.

If I were just eight years older, I could just retire. I guess it's good that I'm not because I would really be tempted. Then what would I do? I would just have more time to miss you. Oh, how I miss you. I would love to say, "Welcome back, Cj. We missed you so much." So, what do I do, Cj? I know. I feel the pain, experience the sorrow, grieve, heal a little and grow a little. Sometimes I get tired of the lessons and just want to curl into a ball and roll away.

I read that grief will go on for years. Is that really so? Will there be many more showers of tears? So, far I feel blessed that I have not had to go through many rivers of tears. There seem to be intermittent showers and sprinkles and clouds and occasional sunshine. I think I will look for the sun when it shines. I forget to focus on the times that I actually feel good during each day. You were and are the sunshine of my life. I will look for you in the beautiful things and know you are smiling at me. I will look for you in the daffodils that are just beginning to bloom. I will look for you in the blossoms of the acacia trees. I will look for you across a beautiful view on a clear day. I will look for you in your sister's loving eyes. I will look for you in your father's warm embrace. I will feel your spirit surrounding me. However, I will miss your human presence.

I love you so much and always will. Thank you for helping me with this letter. I will write again when I am feeling really blue.

With loving memory, Mom

Twenty-four

Cj Writes Back

Only a day had passed since I journaled the letter to Cj. Time seemed to go so slow. Once again I sat down at the computer and journaled.

021200

I have felt such pain and sorrow over the past couple of days. I realized it began late in the afternoon exactly three weeks after Cj's passing. I cry more often although still intermittently. I read that grief is the way we slowly cut the ties that bind us to the physical presence of the person who passed over. Also, I realized that if Cj had gone on a vacation, three weeks would be long enough. I would really be missing her by now. I am experiencing "Missing Her." It is the sense of missing her that immediately fills my eyes with tears. Last night, I was watching an old movie that had been filmed in the Carlsbad Caverns. It hurt to know that we would never be able to take Cj to see those caverns. We always loved exploring caverns together as a family.

I realized that we would never be able to take Cj anywhere with us again. Whenever Chuck and I went somewhere without the girls we would say, "We must come back here and show this place to them." We had dreams of places that we wanted to take them. We had not seen the Grand Canyon together. However, Chuck and I had already realized that if we took the girls everywhere we went for the first time we would not be able to afford to go to all the places of our dreams. Deep in my mind I know Cj is with me, and she will be accompanying me to all these places. However, another part of me does not believe this, and I feel great pain that she is not here. I had read that when I feel really sad I can ask my loved one to write to me. Help me, Cj, and write to me through my fingertips. I began to write this response from Cj.

Oh, Mom,

I know you are feeling great pain, sorrow and grief. I am right beside you, but you cannot see me. When in pain you cannot feel my presence. Each time you feel pain you will slowly learn not to touch areas that are hot, just as a child learns not to touch the hot stove. Few people on this earth have received training in predicting and comprehending the emotions that arise following the passing of a loved one. Therefore, learning occurs through experience like touching a hot stove. Certain thoughts bring pain while other thoughts bring joy. This has been the natural way of learning for millenniums. Few understand this process. You are told that you have to go through stages of mourning, that these feelings will go back and forth, and these feelings are natural and acceptable. But why do you have to go through them?

You thought that since you looked for the lesson in each experience that you might be spared the pain of my passing. You intellectually understand the reasons for my passing and what you can do to benefit mankind through your experiences. You keep busy. This way of coping is beneficial. However, you must also go through the pain. You must experience the heartache. You do not have to analyze everything and consciously learn from it. Believe it or not, that is a limited way of learning. You only have so much conscious brainpower. You learned that only twelve percent of the brain works on the conscious level while eighty-eight percent works on the subconscious level. If you try to rationalize everything, learning will be limited.

This is why feelings are so important. They touch the subconscious mind, which is so powerful in learning. Most people fear their feelings, especially those they consider to be negative. These are the feelings that make you uncomfortable. You do not like these feelings, and you want to avoid them. However, maybe once again you have things backwards. Are these feelings really negative? Remember, "negative" is a judgement. What you might consider negative another person might consider positive. Some people hate to feel angry while others enjoy the feeling of anger. It is much better not to judge the feeling and just realize that you are feeling something. When that feeling is painful it is educating your subconscious mind.

Sometimes the painful feelings may be suggesting that where you are is not the best place for you right now. That does not mean that you deny the feeling. Rather you recognize it, call it by name and say, "This situation (or thought) makes me feel _____." Take responsibility for your feelings, and do not blame them on others. It is less wise to say, "He is insensitive because he does not acknowledge my sorrow," than to say, "I feel sad when he does not offer any words of concern." Your feelings are your feelings. Do not judge the person or situation for causing your feelings. The cause comes from deep within you and provides you the opportunity for growth.

So, dearest Mother, you will have pain because of my passing. Your pain shows you how much you loved me and how much you continue to love me. You also learned to love all others so deeply. You joined all others in the world who have experienced one of mankind's greatest sorrows — the loss of one's child. Your pain will slowly lessen as you learn subconsciously not to touch the "hot areas." It is only natural to touch these areas now because they are all that you know. However, as time passes your subconscious mind will go to the areas that are not "hot" but to those that bring joy. When you think of me with a sense of joy I will be with you. You can sense that I'm am with you if you choose to be aware. Without the pain, you would stay attached to my physical memory. By releasing those memories you will soar with me among the heavens.

> I love all of you,
> *Cj*

Twenty-five

"Hi" to My Dad

It was Sunday morning, and I felt more peaceful than I had felt in days. I knew that Cj's letter had helped me understand and accept my pain. In many ways I found it hard to watch Chuck going through his pain in his own way. He had not written anything since the day before Cj passed away. He seemed to be trapped in such pain and sorrow. I was checking my e-mail and then felt led to open Chuck's e-mail address. I began to type this letter.

021300

"Hi" to my blessed Dad,

As you know, I can chat with you through Mom. I love you so very much. I know that you can feel my loving energy around you. You know why I had to change form. I had to be free from being restricted to the body and explode out to be with all people that I love. There is a lot of joyful work that needs to be done. I love you so much and cradle you often in my arms. Sometimes I use Mom's arms to cradle you, and she often knows when this is happening.

You and Mom make such a great team together. You have no idea what you are going to be up to. I know that you are going through pain right now. I told Mom that it is like an amputation. It takes time for the pain to heal. Often I talk to you through Mom. You told Mom that there will always be a void because I am gone and that the same is true when your father passed away when you were fifteen. Mom's words were right about not having to have a void. That is old programming and part of the philosophy of the Western culture. Many people felt such a void from the loss of money during the depression that they actually jumped out of windows. That void did not have to be there.

The mind identifies the heart's pain as emptiness. However, it is what it is — pain. Pain from loss does not have to be rationalized as anything else. It is pain. The pain lessens in time, and a great joy can replace it. This great joy can also be accompanied by great power. You could not love Mom as you do right now if you did not have similar awareness. Without this, you and Mom would have become opposites. The opposite polarities would have caused friction. Your awareness was growing along with hers, but neither of you knew it. Mom was beginning to suspect. You have a beautiful gift that you can develop if you let go of your fear.

I am with you always. Even when you do not think of me I am with you. I love you. I know that you have to go through this time of great sadness. Mom also knows and trusts that you will be okay. I know that you will be okay. The cycle repeats itself: pain, sorrow, grief, healing and then growth. You and Mom have grown so much. There is beautiful work to be done.

I cradle you. I love you. I embrace you with my loving energy. Sit quietly and think of me. Think of me as that baby that you cradled in your arms. I will wink at you and tell you some stories. I love to tell stories. Sit quietly. Breathe and count each breath going in. Breathe and count each breath going out. Breathe and count each breath, in and out, up to twenty (in as number one and out as two). Then just relax and empty your mind. Ask me a question, and I will answer through your thoughts. I will answer questions, or I can just tell you a story. Ask whatever you would like.

I love you, my blessed father. I cherish what I learned from you at earth school. Listen quietly and I can share those lessons with you.

Until later,

Your blessed daughter, young spirit, old soul, up-to-something,

Cj

Twenty-six

Moments of Now

We celebrated my mother's birthday on February 17. My whole family was together — except Cj. We tried to make everything light-hearted; we tried to celebrate life. However, I was watching my mother, and something was missing. She looked tired. She had been so strong during Cj's illness even though her heart was weak. I did not know what I sensed, but I felt sad. That night, I journaled this poem, and my burden lifted enough for me to go to bed.

Moments of Now

The toughest moments in my life are those of now, not
    yesterday.
Past memories can bring joy and smiles upon my face.
Past hurts dissolve into fairy dust that scatters in the wind.
Future hopes are for peace and a light-heartedness free
    from sorrow.
Future quests are for a glowing Love for all mankind.

The toughest moments in my life are those of now, not
    yesterday.
It is right now that I feel the pain of sorrow and
    insecurity.

The ache was absent a minute ago, but now knocks at my
heart.
I feel my pain; I feel my sorrow; I feel my loss. I touch It.
I touch It and my body quivers; I gasp and shed some
tears.

The toughest moments in my life are those of now, not
yesterday.
It is now that the tears glisten, the taste of salt reminding
me of earth's cycles.
The tears of now tell me that I am one with all through
sorrow.
My ache draws my thoughts within, drifting from
resentful to empowered.
I wonder at the universal process: Loss bringing pain,
sorrow, healing and growth.

The toughest moments in my life are those of now, not
yesterday.
My opportunities for insights, choices, decisions and
action are now.
The lessons, if I saw and heard, grew out of many
yesterdays.
The future holds a reward for me each time a part of me
has healed.
I feel, I touch, I heal, and I grow in the moments of now,
not yesterday.

Twenty-seven

Tears

Chuck and I were listening to music from *The Phantom of the Opera* while coming home from a three-year-old child's birthday party. The song "Music of the Night" brought tears to my eyes as I remembered taking the kids to see *The Phantom*. I thought about how we would never go to another play or musical with Cj again. The song reminded me of Cj listening to her music in the hospital and how I would put on a CD for her each night before I left. I realized that this is another concept that hurts: the "Never Agains." I knew the "Never Agains" were very similar to the "What Might Have Beens" and that both were not the best places to remain. I felt my tears sting my cheeks. At first, I was self-conscious that I was crying and concerned that Chuck would notice and worry about me. Then I relaxed and reminded myself to breathe.

I felt the tears flowing down my cheeks. I thought about what I was feeling. I tried to touch the actual emotion and realized that once again the pain lessened. Not only did the pain soon leave, but I did not have any strong feelings. I thought, "Why am I so concerned about my tears? Do I really know what they signify, or am I so conditioned to trying to avoid them that I have no knowledge regarding their purpose?" Again I went within and felt no pain. I just let the tears flow and my nose run.

I did not even bother to wipe them. When they stopped, I was not aware that I felt any different than before the tears started. I did not think I had felt stressed before I began listening to the music, and I did not feel stressed after crying. What was the purpose of those tears? Later that evening I wrote an e-mail to a friend about the tears. The next morning I re-read the e-mail and received some insights. I opened my journal and wrote about my tears.

022000

Yesterday, we went to a birthday party at Cj's godparents' house. The party was for their grandchild, Shelby, and the house was filled with young children and young parents. It was my first social outing since Cj's passing. Some acquaintances were there who knew we had lost Cj. However, many of the younger parents had no idea, and I shared my experiences about Cj's illness and passing with just a few. Elise and I spent most of our time sitting on the couch holding hands while watching the toddlers and babies. One young mother asked me if Elise was my baby. I had already learned that similar questions could bring on a sudden sense of shock. I felt shock, pain, and experienced sorrow and grief the first time someone asked me how many children I had. I was more prepared this time. I patted Elise's hand and just answered, "Yes."

What about the tears that flowed last night while I listened to the music? I do not know where they came from or why I was crying. I have learned not to fight them. I have learned to let the tears flow, not to judge them and not to judge myself for crying. Last night, I refused to fear the tears or fear touching the pain that might lurk behind them. I was rewarded once again. I tried to touch the feeling and realized that the pain floated away. But, I did not discover the lesson last night when I wrote the e-mail.

My lesson came to me this morning while thinking about my tears. I had no idea I had been feeling pain and sorrow all day at the birthday party. I was again playing the part of the stoic mother when it came to the pain of the loss of a child. I was not comfortable crying at work in front of my co-workers or patients. In no way would I allow myself to cry at Shelby's birthday party. There is a time to weep and a time to refrain from weeping. There is a time to weep. That is my lesson.

There were many times after Cj became ill and after her passing that there was no time to weep. I wept at her bedside on Tuesday, two days before she passed. I thought I was mourning. Do I, or any of us, really know what mourning is? I remember telling the nurse in the room in Intensive Care that I never had a chance to mourn Cj since she became ill. I wept. There had never been a time to weep before; not in front of her when she was alert, not driving home, not in front of my family, nor at work. The time had finally arrived on that Tuesday night, and I wept. I wept while touching her and on the way home. That evening we wept together as a family: Chuck, Elise and I in each other's arms.

I had not reflected on the tears. I had reflected on the pain, but not the tears. I realized after the birthday party that the tears helped to heal the hidden pain that I had been experiencing throughout the duration of the party. I had even hidden the pain from myself. It was the music that triggered the tears. My thoughts of loss helped them flow. My acceptance of the tears kept them flowing until the healing from that painful situation was complete. The tears are part of the grief process. I had often read and heard that tears release tension and stress and that those who cry suffer less from stress than those that don't cry. I knew that intellectually. Last night I accepted my tears. I went "with the flow." I did not fight or judge them. Today I reflected on tears and learned a beauti-ful lesson. Tears are magic. They are a gift to be treasured.

Twenty-eight

The Thank You Letter

We received many beautiful bouquets of flowers for Cj's memorial service. The bouquet that lasted the longest was the one that came from the Big Island of Hawaii. We had visited Hawaii the month before Cj got sick. In February, 1999, she begged for a Hawaiian family vacation. We managed to go, and while we were there we visited an old friend of mine, Michael. We used to work together years ago, and I had not seen him for over fifteen years. Cj met him for the first time when we visited his home in Hawaii, and they bonded right away.

It took me about a month to write and thank him for the flowers. I had never been able to tell Michael about Cj's illness and passing. He found out from mutual friends of ours, Cj's godparents. I knew that the thank-you had to be more that just a short note. I would have to touch what had happened once again and had not been ready to re-live the pain. This thank-you letter became a journal entry

030700

Dear Michael,

I am sorry that it has taken me so long to write. The flowers you sent were beautiful. It is the only bouquet remaining; it still has a few of the flowers and leaves. Your flowers came two days before Cj's memorial service, so I left them in the box. On the day of the service, I arranged them at the church, and they were perfect. We put them right next to the memory board that displayed pictures of Cj growing up.

For some reason my intuition said that the fellowship room (where we held the service) had to be decorated in teal. I could not figure out why. While I was arranging your Hawaiian flowers a thought came to me, "The color is not teal, it is aqua. It symbolizes the Age of Aquarius." I know that Cj's passing has something to do with the Age of Aquarius. Your flowers also represented the Age of Aquarius. Her illness and death touched many people — children, friends, parents, the medical field and therapists. Over 250 people attended the memorial service. We were amazed to hear how Cj had touched so many people's lives, even if only with just her smile.

I do not believe in chance. I saw too many miracles during Cj's illness. Even Kaiser Hospital's activity director, Pat, chose to go to the places in Hawaii that Cj had described to her. She was on the bay (by the Captain Cook Monument) about the time Cj passed away. Pat called back to the Kaiser nurses in Oakland to say that the spinner dolphins had been jumping all over the place. I believe the dolphins were celebrating. When Chuck and I went back to Kaiser to visit the nurses, they showed us the last room Cj had occupied before she went to ICU at Children's Hospital. Kaiser had put up a wallpaper border around the top of the wall. The design was of a colorful underwater scene of a person snorkeling with beautiful tropical fish. The border went up right after Cj vacated the room. The nurses said they believe Cj had a hand in it and that all the children's rooms are going to have this border. A few days later, I turned over a post card that was on our coffee table. It was a dolphin. My intuitive thought was, "Cj's totem is the dolphin."

We were encouraged by friends, physicians and social workers to share how we dealt with Cj's illness and passing. We did not think we had done anything differently, but we did not have any past experiences or precedents to guide us. We used love, compassion and humor. We were told that other families just did not deal with life threatening illness that way. They did not decorate rooms nor share what they were learning from each situation. My intuition told me that I would be writing a book called *The Healing Room*. So, throughout Cj's illness I was looking for the healing room (the hospital room, home, etc.). I also received an e-mail from a friend early during Cj's illness. It included a story about Rumi, a thirteenth century poet, catching Grief drinking from the cup of sorrow and saying, "Ah, how joyful." Rumi said, "I caught you." Grief said, "Now, you have ruined it for me. How can I sell sorrow when you know it's such a blessing?" So with each cup of sorrow during Cj's illness, her passing and afterwards, I looked for the lesson that brings joy. A big message of the book will be not to fear sorrow, but to experience it as a natural part of being human. Some of the greatest healing comes from sorrow. The healing room is in the heart and soul.

We also decided that one of the best ways to try to share our experience and help others is to start a foundation. As you know from your loss, it keeps one busy and helps give meaning to the passing of someone we love. We hope to call it the CJ Foundation. Its mission will be to lessen the anguish of families experiencing life threatening illness and/or the death of a loved one through education and charitable giving. One goal is to start helping to merge alternative holistic therapies with Western medicine. For Cj, we were able to include acupressure, aromatherapy, energy, crystals, and music. This gave us something to contribute, to do and gave us hope.

So again, thank you for the beautiful flowers. I still reflect on how interesting it is that Cj chose to go to Hawaii for her last vacation and had the chance to meet you. I don't know if she was saying goodbye, hello or both. Maybe you both had secret gifts for each other.

Let's keep in touch.
Love, Dori

Twenty-nine

Finding Peace

My seventy-four-year-old mother has had congestive heart failure for many years. She stayed very strong during Cj's illness and often drove my dad (who had recently broken his back) to the hospital to visit Cj. However, Cj's death caused further weakening of my mother's heart and health. One month after Cj passed away, and three days after my mother's birthday, I received news from the primary nurse that my mother was quite ill. The nurse told me that we should appreciate every moment with her. I asked how long we could expect her to live. The nurse said that was unknown; however, our mother did not have long.

I went over regularly to help fix meals and, at times, stayed and ate with my parents. All my sisters were helping. The whole family went out for dinner with Mom and Dad three Sundays in a row. My mother seemed to improve. She seemed to be breathing and thinking better and was even preparing meals. However, her legs were swollen, so we helped put on wet compresses.

I went over after work to put the compresses on Mom's legs. Dad had been doing it several times during the day and his back ached. I know we were all concerned about Mom's health and were tired. I got into a brief argument with my father. This was very significant for me because I had never yelled at my father before. It hurt, but a part of me grew and healed after I journaled.

032300

My mother is not doing well because of heart failure. Her mind is pretty good, but her legs are swollen and she is weak. I went over last evening and during lunch today to put the compresses on her legs. We were using warm towels. I noticed that the towels were new and old ones were hanging over the shower door to dry. My father got very angry when I mentioned that the towels might develop bacteria in them if not put in the washer. I got angry at the way he responded. I was saying I liked the new towels and it would allow the others to be washed. I did not put up with his outburst. I told him to stop acting like a two-year-old. He said he would if people stopped treating him like one. This was the first time in my forty-eight years that I did not silently accept my father's angry outbursts. My father stomped out of the room. My mother spoke to me gently and lovingly. She said, "I bet you feel better." I said, "No, not really. I hate getting angry." Besides I felt guilty. Wisely she said, " But you do feel better, now."

That evening I called Charlee about the towels, and she called the Heart Clinic. She called me back and said that we are not to worry about the bacteria. Mom's doctor said that there is nothing much more that can be done. Mom's heart just cannot pump the fluids. Just keep putting on the compresses.

Mom told me last night that her doctor said she was worried about her. I sat down with Mom and asked her how she felt. She said, "Worried." We talked about the after-life and that if there really is one then it sounds like a wonderful place. I believe we all worry about dying or else we would not stay here. However, maybe there comes a time when worrying is no longer needed. Maybe there comes a time when we can just enjoy our final days and not try to learn any more life lessons. Maybe we can just peacefully reflect on all that has happened throughout our life and about what we have learned and not attend any more classes. Maybe we get to watch people scurrying around still trying to figure out what it is all about.

Maybe we can gather in all our experiences and look at the picture that we painted, the tapestry that we wove, and the grand puppet show in which we were the stars. Maybe we earn a break if we lived our life to our best ability, trying to do that which we thought would help, trying to learn to love, and trying to learn to forgive ourselves. Maybe we earn the opportunity to be at peace, free from anxiety and free from worry. We just have to accept that opportunity. We just have to accept the offering of free will. We can choose to continue to worry about the "Might Have Beens" and the "What Might Happens" or we can choose to be in the moment. We can choose fear or we can choose faith. We can choose resentment or choose acceptance. Maybe it's an ultimate choice between peace and struggle. If so, I choose Peace.

Thirty

Hope and Faith

I talked to the cardiac nurse again to find out how my mother was doing. The nurse said Home Health Hospice had been recommended. I knew that meant my mother had less than six months to live. Mom said she did not want Home Health. That made sense for now because she was able to do things for herself. Mom called me Sunday night to say that her doctor had told her that there was not much more that the medical field could do for her. She had told me this previously, but I don't think she remembered. I do not think I thought about the impact either.

After the nurse called I began thinking about what would happen after my mother was gone. I wanted to have many moments with her before she left. My life continued to be disrupted, or at least was not what I would have chosen if my mother was not ill. However, I did not want to experience any regrets after she passed away. My mother and I even spoke about death together for the first time in our lives. I shared my thought, "If it is as beautiful on the other side as those who have seen the light say, then why would we be anxious and fearful?" If there is nothing on the "other side" then being anxious or fearful is not going to help either. I do believe that we need a certain amount of fear of death or else, maybe, we would not be willing to stay on earth and go through all the pain it offers. I knew I would be facing an additional pain soon. I had been hurting, so I turned to my journal.

032900

I felt very sad on Monday and Tuesday. However, the sadness was no heavier than when Cj passed away. I believe that there is a threshold for sadness, and it can't get any worse. Sadness is just sadness. I did notice that it came around more often. I cried a little longer and cried a little more in front of other people. I even took a day off from work. I had a sense of feeling lost. I had a sense of feeling resigned to the inevitable — my mother's heart weakening day by day. I felt helpless. I felt hopeless. At times, some family members, including myself, became irritated and said things to each other that we did not really mean. I talked to the nurse again and wanted to know how long we had with my mother. Again she said that my mother was in the end stage of heart failure and that she did not have long. I asked, "Just between you and me, can you give me an idea of how long she has?" The nurse said, "No, I'm sorry, I can't." I felt discouraged.

The next day I realized I was experiencing the hopelessness and loss of faith that others felt during Cj's illness. I had refused to lose hope for Cj, but hopelessness crept up on me with my mother's illness. I realized that once again I wanted to be in control. Just like I wanted to know if the ventilator could be stopped so we could know when Cj would pass, I wanted to know when my mother would pass. I had learned to give up control during Cj's illness and passing. However, I tried to take control back again when it came to my mother's illness. My desire for control only caused me to feel hopeless, helpless, lost, irritable, and discouraged. I smiled and said, "Alright, I give up control. I never really had it in the first place, and it only causes me greater grief."

On Tuesday, my mother saw a cardiologist. The cardiologist told her that he still felt there were some medications to try. My mother said, "He seems to have more hope for me than my other doctor does." My mother is going to try another medication. All of a sudden a burden lifted from my shoulders. Then I realized the lesson. When I try to take control I only have hope and faith in myself. However, I have no ability to cure my mother's heart, to lessen her discomfort, nor to stop the cycle of birth and death. Nor do I have the right to know when my mother's time, or anyone's time for passing over, will come. If I want control over other people's situations then I ask for hopelessness. I do not have control. Control is an illusion.

I gave up control of my mother's illness to her medical team. I decided to choose hope and faith in their judgements, leadership and recommendations. I decided to reject control and welcome hope and faith in the cycle of life and death. I have faith that whatever happens is the way it is supposed to be. I have hope and faith that my mother will be more comfortable and peaceful. I have hope and faith that I can spend our time together with me as her daughter and not her watchdog or mentor. I have hope and faith that I can learn from her by being silent and listening to her or by listening to my answers when she asks me questions.

I release control to the wind. I release its burden from my shoulders. I welcome Hope and Faith as they replace control. I welcome the gift of joy that comes from Hope and Faith.

Thirty-one

The Drawer

Over two months had passed since Cj's death, and I rarely went into her room. Occasionally, I went in to store something under her bed or in the closet. The floor was a mess. It was covered with all the tangled-up deflated balloons, paper bags full of toys, games and books that were at the hospital, pink plastic basins full of medical supplies, and the linens and comforters that we had bought for her bed at the hospital. I had not been able to spend time in her room because it was too painful. Then I found myself looking for my little brass hammer.

Where did my special hammer go? I hadn't seen it for months. It is a brass hammer with a set of screwdrivers inside the handle. It was not in any of the likely or unlikely places. Where could my hammer possibly be? Suddenly, I thought about how Cj loved to nail things to her walls and how she had even created a little shelf all by herself. She rarely returned the tools that she used. The hammer might be in her room. If I wanted the hammer I would have to look in Cj's room. I knew it would be a very painful experience. However, I had learned that a wonderful insight always followed pain when I took the time to reflect upon and journal the experience. I wrote this after finding the hammer.

040100

 I had not been able to find my little brass hammer for some time. I finally suspected that it was in Cj's room. I knew I would have to look for it in her drawers. During my search, I noticed that her drawers were all organized according to make-up, hair items, socks, pens and pencils, pajamas, shirts, etc. This neatness was a little surprising, as she tended to leave things very cluttered. Each drawer gently tugged on my heart as my hand swept over the items. Then I opened a bottom drawer and felt that familiar stab of pain. I sat down cross-legged and pulled the drawer onto the floor. It was her Drawer. It was the Treasure Drawer.

The first things that I found were my hammer and two pairs of pliers. I smiled and shook my head at how often she had taken our things to her room but became so upset if we used something of hers. I started sorting through the drawer and tears began streaming down my cheeks. I wailed out loud and rocked myself as I touched the empty gum wrappers, the tiny broken toys, the candy wrappers, the broken pieces of jewelry, the bottle tops, the iridescent stickers, the audio-tapes, and old game pieces. I wailed for the human being that had been my child.

It is natural to idealize the dead, especially when one has passed away early in life. I can idealize our daughter, say that it was all meant to be and refuse to remember that she was a human being. I can choose to forget that her physical presence was such an important part of our family. By forgetting, I can dull that pain and even paint over it with rainbow colors of martyrdom.

I decided to touch her Drawer. I touched the pain and sorrow and let the tears stream down my face. Then I was surrounded by peace and began to reflect. Her Drawer reminded me that Cj was a human being just like all the rest of us. Most people I know have a Treasure Drawer that expresses the cluttered aspects of our lives. However, this is the Drawer that most of us keep secret. I realized I even have more than one. One is a drawer and one is a shelf in my closet. Until now, I would have been embarrassed if someone rummaged through my treasure spots. Now I realize that my Treasure Drawer is what shows me that I am human. In all my attempts to be organized, I do not give up my Treasure Drawer. I may take out some items I no longer need, but I always seem to put another thing in.

Cj's Drawer helped me to remember that she was human. She is my child who I will always ache to hold. I also am human. There will be days when I look into my organized drawers and remember Cj in an ideal way. There will be those days when I open my Treasure Drawer and reminiscence about the days gone by. However, I am learning that both drawers remind me that I am able to feel. Knowing that I do feel tells me that am alive. I am alive and am going to feel all that this world has to offer.

Thirty-two

Energy Loss from Addictions

I had been gaining weight and didn't feel motivated to do anything about it. I had watched my weight, almost too carefully, since I was a teenager. I was fearful of getting heavy. My fear came from family conditioning because my mother had been heavy until her heart failure. When she was heavy she would point out other people who were heavy, especially if they were eating. Now, for the first time in my life I did not care about my weight. Instead of watching the scale I began to watch my habits. One day I felt the urge to write.

040400

Since Cj has passed away I find myself eating more sweets, craving salty chips and watching more television. On my way home from work I make myself a promise that I will not eat any sweets or chips before or after dinner. Regularly, by the time I walk into the kitchen I am heading for the cookie jar or the bag of chips. I sit down at the television instead of writing, reading that book, going for a walk or even just taking a short nap. If the sweets are so hard to give up then they must be some kind of addiction. After I eat them I do not feel better; I have less energy. This makes me think of addictions.

I think of addictions as behaviors that keep me from looking at the situation that is causing my energy loss, the reasons for this loss and the lessons I could be learning. Addictions replace my pain and sorrow. Addictions prevent me from going through the grieving process. Addictions interfere with my ability to learn lessons from life. Addiction results from avoidance and can be avoidance, itself. Addictions drain my energy and interfere with my healing.

If I lose my energy, I lose my life force, my peacefulness, and then I lose joy. This loss of joy is powerful when I use it as a barometer for how I am doing in life. How am I approaching life's lessons? If I remain angry or fearful then most likely I am using avoidance and that avoidance is an addiction. The addiction may give a sudden sense of contentment or even a rush, but it is temporary. The fear and anger will return quickly. Then I have to turn to that addictive behavior again to be content.

There are many addictions. Society in general recognizes drugs to be addicting, whether legal or not. Many say that we need a war on drugs and for the children just to say no. How can one go to war with something that is not alive? Can we make war with alcohol, cigarettes, syringes, and pills? They can't even fight back. How does one go to war against something that cannot fight back? If a war were started with something that could not fight back, wouldn't the aggressor win immediately? Everyone could flush alcohol, cigarettes and pills down the toilet and the war would be over. Why hasn't the war against drugs been won?

I wonder if the battle needs to be against the avoidance of feelings. It would be silly for me to start a war on sweets and chips. I don't think the supermarkets would like it anyway. To beat the addictions we need to feel. I believe I am willing to feel the pain from the loss of Cj. I know I feel the pain, I cry,

I mourn and then I accept her passing once again. But I also know that when I sit down and do the exact thing that I promised myself that I would not do, I am avoiding my feelings. How can I learn from my feelings and discover what I really want to do if I avoid the feelings that are trying to surface because I am doing what I do not really want to do?

Thirty-three

Let It Be

It was a Friday and had been a typical day at work. I shared information about energy and the life force with a group of patients. I demonstrated how identifying our feelings actually raises our energy and makes us feel better. Judging another person or a situation causes our energy to drop. I demonstrated how saying, "Cancel, cancel!" raises one's energy by counteracting the negative thought. All who tried it agreed that they felt lighter and less burdened after thinking, " Cancel." Then I remembered that being perplexed or in a quandary also caused energy to drop. I have spent a lot of time wondering about my life since Cj's death. I have been spending a lot of time in quandary and have not been using the technique of canceling my perplexed thoughts. I journaled my thoughts during lunch.

040700

At some point we understand that we do not have to analyze every situation. I know when my buttons are pushed. I am aware of what my basic triggers are. I have learned to step back after getting angry and think about my lesson. I do not always like the fact that there is someone there to teach me another lesson by pushing my button, but I also understand that the person is a mirror to myself.

There are times to analyze and times to refrain from analyzing. I know that when I am in a quandary my energy level is lower. If I go around trying to analyze myself every time I feel my cheeks burn then my energy will be lower. I do not have to know everything about myself. I can let it go. I can just learn to be. The key for me is "back to basics." I taught the basics this morning. I taught the thoughts "cancel" and "I feel." These two thoughts are powerful in raising my energy level.

It is difficult to let go of my defenses while dealing with people. I do not have to fully analyze my defenses. Also, my defenses may be there for reasons that I do not really understand. I may only think I have figured them out. How much easier it would be to use "cancel" and "I feel" when experiencing an uncomfortable situation. When I try to analyze my discomfort I am distracted from the speaker. Also, the energy level between us is lowered. When I think the words "I feel" and "cancel," the signal fails to trigger my defenses, and I can concentrate on what is actually happening or being said. I can let it be.

It is not easy to let it be. I want to change the world. I want others to be like me, to experience my joy, to have my insights, to do it my way, etc. I know that is not possible and is unrealistic. However, maybe it has been very difficult for part of me to get past being a two-year-old. Two-year-olds want everything their way. We are all unique, and each of us must go through life differently. I went to a support group last night and truly discovered how each loss and how one handles it is unique. Part of me said, "Just listen" and part of me said, "Tell them there is another way." I did a lot of listening. We must go through our own pain and hopefully experience our own grief and sorrow if we are willing. I will try to let it be for others as well as myself.

By asking, "Why?" I have discovered the reasons for having to go through my tragic experience. After my tears I often experienced insights that helped me heal and grow as a person. I still cry. I still receive insights, but I am becoming more content to just let it be. Maybe this is acceptance.

Thirty-four

Loss

I had checked the mail and there was a letter from the county assessor's office. We had added on to our home in 1995, and I filled out all the paperwork for re-assessing taxes. However, we never received a tax increase on our bill. I knew I had completed the forms, so we did not do anything about it. Each year the tax bill came, and there was no increase. Now the letter had come. Now an assessor wanted to come and re-assess our home. I went into a panic. I remained upset all day even though Chuck assured me there was nothing to worry about and that he would work with the assessor. I knew I needed to journal the experience since I was so upset.

041200

I experienced fear, apprehension and anxiety last evening. There was a notice in the mail from the assessor regarding assessing our new addition. In retrospect it felt like a mild panic attack. Fortunately, Chuck came home soon after I read the notice.

The problem, as I saw it, was that taxes had not been levied on our 1995 addition. Chuck was amazingly calm. I have such a great deal of respect for how he does not react to things. I reflected on my fear. I realized that I had never mourned losing my childhood home in Crow Canyon when the road was widened. I always said that it was my parents' loss and that I learned through observation. I realized that I had never mourned. I had denied that the loss of my home, my friends, my horse, and my high school had any effect on me. I remember saying that I looked forward to the change and was tired of caring for a horse.

We moved up north to a small town. My father took a leave of absence from teaching and bought a dry cleaning business. I was fifteen when we moved. I knew no one except my brother. My brother and I had to work at the cleaners after school and on alternate Saturdays. At first, I did not have any friends and remember focusing on my life in the San Francisco Bay Area. I was the studious type who grew friends slowly. In a couple of months I had made some friends and had some fun and memorable times. In the middle of my sophomore year I had a boyfriend who was a senior. He left in late summer to be an exchange student in Germany, and I did not mourn my loss. I rationalized the loss. I read the poem "Absence is to love what wind is to fire; it extinguishes the little and kindles the big." I rationalized that this absence was a test of our relationship. I stayed loyal and did not date my junior year. I befriended an exchange student from Norway. She left at the end of my junior year. I did not mourn the loss of her friendship. I rationalized that it was what I knew would happen when I met her. My motto by age seventeen was to "keep a stiff upper lip."

I was busy the summer before my senior year. I knew we were moving back to the San Francisco Bay Area. I did not write and tell my boyfriend that I would be moving. I was visiting the Bay Area when he returned home from Germany, and according to my parents, he drove to my house, and discovered them packing. I had one more date with him.

I lost his friendship (if I ever had it) because I had not been honest. I did not mourn that loss. I blamed myself for not being honest. I rationalized the lesson.

We moved back to the Bay Area. My father resumed teaching and was assigned to Castlemont High in Oakland. I did an out-of-district transfer and went to Castlemont High with Dad. It provided a great life lesson, and making friends was easy. I had three girlfriends at school (the only other girls of my race). When I graduated I did not maintain the friendships. I realize now that for years I did not maintain any close friendships. I did not allow anyone to get close. I did not allow myself to need people. I still don't. I've wondered whether throughout my life I really knew what Love was. Did I protect myself from loving out of fear of experiencing loss? Did I fool myself that I loved? If I really did love would I have gotten so angry when I felt overwhelmed or unappreciated? Does this have anything to do with never having mourned the loss of a home, friends, and a way of life, but rationalizing the losses instead?

Today, I enjoy being with friends, entertaining, going out to dinner, talking, or playing cards. However, I always find myself reluctant to commit to getting together. Often others have to make the first contact. I do not like to be with people for extended periods of time. I do not like to commit to getting together, especially if I do not feel I will have time alone or the freedom to be alone. I do not feel comfortable if friends begin to need me. I do not know if this is the way it needs to be or if it is an area I need to grow in. I love my family. I felt removed from my extended family but have always loved my husband and children dearly. They have been my greatest teachers in learning how to love. I have always wanted them near me. I loved Cj dearly and lost her.

I lost my home at fifteen. I have never been comfortable with a nice home. For many years I managed to keep my home in a state of limbo with unfinished construction projects. In 1995, my home was remodeled, with me voting against the project. Now the home is beautiful. I do love it. I have worked so hard not to be proud of it as "pride comes before a fall." The re-assessment was looming. Now I am once again facing the possibility of loss. I am not sure what kind of loss, but the possibility disturbs me. I cannot even handle the situation. Chuck was so calm about taking care of the whole thing.

I believe with Cj's illness and death that I am finally learning to look at things differently. I know that I must feel my fears, acknowledge them and touch them. I am not alone in this situation. Whatever happens with the house, I will mourn, if necessary. I will feel the pain and the grief that may follow. I know it will pass. It will be nothing compared to what we continue to go through over Cj's passing. As Chuck said, it is only a thing. It is only money. Things can be fixed. Money is available. We have very little control over health.

Maybe there is an underlying wound in my heart and soul that never healed because I did not recognize it was there. How can I know all the wounds that exist? Some may go back very far. To move on, to grow as a person, the wounds of the heart and soul must be healed and the scars removed. They cannot just be erased as if nothing ever happened. Life continues, lessons reveal themselves and I heal when I feel, mourn and grieve. Then I learn from the experience. To do this I must accept responsibility for my own experiences, not blame others, but look for the meaning that lies within. Then I heal and grow. Then I am ready to face the next lesson that waits around the bend. Maybe over time I will learn to celebrate these opportunities to grow rather than seeing them as unfair burdens placed upon me.

Thirty-five

The Seasons

One Saturday morning, I was walking around the house doing simple chores. I felt periodic waves of pressure on my chest and in my heart. Occasionally, my eyes welled up with tears, and at other times I found myself smiling. I cried when I looked at a picture of Cj. In many ways I understood why Cj passed away so young. I saw the direct positive impact her death had on others. Many people, including Elise's teenage friends, seemed to appreciate life much more. Even so, I ached for Cj. I wrote to her.

041500

Dear Cj,

My heart is heavy today. My intuitions about the reasons for your passing continue to be confirmed. While this brings me joy, it also brings me such grief. Sometimes I feel like I am going too fast, and sometimes I feel like I am going so slowly. My heart aches.

You came to teach so much to so many. I hope we learned. I hope I can continue to grow and learn to embrace life. I just feel blue today. Elise is going to the Junior Prom. As you know, she is going with your friend, Ben. I just finished taking pictures of them. I guess I am experiencing the "Never Will Be's." Dad and I will never see you go to a prom or a ball. We will never see you date, fall in love or have children. We will never see you again. We will not learn any more lessons from you. You will not correct us when we think in the old way (such as asking what time we'll be heading for home before we even reached our destination). You are gone in form. We will never be a family of four again. We are a family of three. At times this really hurts.

To move on, to learn and grow, there must be loss. That is our greatest lesson. If we learn to experience each loss, to feel the fear, the insecurity, the pain, the grief and release the tears that often accompany loss, we heal and grow. That is the greatest lesson we can learn. When we feel the pain, we can identify with the experience. We cannot identify with other people's experiences unless we've also had a similar experience. We cannot learn without having experiences of loss.

What is it we need to learn? Learning to be grateful brings great joy even for the smallest things in life. Grateful means to love what it is, as it is. We do not learn very well when things are going smoothly. That is not human nature. Some people have learned to be grateful for what they have. However, it is hard to be grateful for something that has always been there. It is easier to be grateful after loss. Sometimes the lesson of loss can come through observing others, listening to the news, watching a movie, etc. Our hearts might ache at the glimpse of wars and people being killed. We are experiencing loss of the illusion that all is well in the world. The pain of seeing others at war helps some of us to be grateful for peace. The pain of seeing someone else tend an ill child or someone else go through the death of a loved one can help make us grateful for health and life. The pain of tending an ill loved one and watching the death process of one so dear provides the opportunity to be grateful for the ability to have loved so much that loss is so painful.

Maybe loss is what Ecclesiastics 3:8 is about. If it is hard to be grateful without loss, then there must be times in our lives when loss is necessary. The cycle of life involves birth and then death, or is the cycle death and then birth? To find something we must first lose something. To experience the joy of life we must experience sorrow. Sorrow comes from war, killing, hatred, tearing down, shunning and death. Gratitude and joy come from peace, healing, love, building up, embracing one another and birth. The experiences are commensurate with each other — the greater the magnitude of the loss, the greater the magnitude of joy. But, the commensurate joy is missed if the loss is not grieved and mourned. Now I understand what Krishnamurti meant when he wrote, "The ending of sorrow is love. To see what is, is to love." The other way of handling loss is to become angry, bitter, resentful and to feel victimized. The lessons of gratitude and compassion are not learned that way. "There is a time to weep and a time to laugh." "Blessed are those who mourn for they shall be comforted." The comfort to the mourner is the great joy that fills the heart from the gratitude of having loved. The greatest of all things is Love.

Thirty-six

Her Music

One Saturday morning Chuck and I were sitting at the table drinking coffee when one of Cj's favorite songs came on the radio. I had already noticed that we had avoided Her Music since she passed away. There were certain new age artists and songs that were special to us as a family. We often listened to music during our travels, and this beautiful music accompanied us during our journey through Cj's illness. We listened to the music in her hospital room, while waiting for her to awake from conscious sedation, and while reading together. Cj shared her favorite rock and roll and "new age" music with the nurses, and they gave Cj suggestions for additional artists that she might enjoy. Also, Cj would request a certain CD to listen to every night at the hospital before I left. That morning, Chuck and I cried through the whole song. I did not realize the impact of this experience until later in the day.

041700

It has been three months since Cj passed away. Chuck and I were having coffee when we heard one of our favorite family songs by Enya on the radio. We began to cry as the familiar pain returned to our chests and throats. We talked about how Cj loved music and how it brought her joy and peace. I noticed that the refrain said, "sail away, sail away, sail away." Sometimes it seems like Cj sailed away. We touched our sorrow and then took each other's hand and smiled.

That afternoon Chuck, Elise and I went to a wedding. The son of very dear friends (Elise's godparents) was getting married. Chuck and I sat there holding hands. We did not even have to talk, but I know we were thinking the same thing. My eyes welled with tears. Then I remembered that every moment in marriage is not blissful, and Cj did not have to go through the ups and downs of learning to love another person unconditionally. She had already learned that lesson.

Suddenly, before the wedding started, the same song by Enya was played. Chuck and I glanced at each other. I was so thankful that we had heard the song earlier on the radio. We had already touched that sorrow and reflected on the joy that comes from music. We did not have to touch our sorrow quite so deeply at the wedding nor break down in tears in front of all those guests. Many of the guests knew that we had lost Cj.

Did Cj send us that song this morning to ease our sorrow so we could touch the joy of a wedding celebration? I think if Chuck and I had refused to listen to the song, feel the pain, and touch our sorrow we would have had even greater pain at the wedding. We did listen to the song. We did feel the pain and sorrow. We touched it without fear and realized what tenderness we have towards each other after sharing so much pain together. The wedding reminded us of our love for each other instead of being an experience of overwhelming loss.

In time, I will be able to listen to more of the music that we loved as a family. Each time I hear this music I will feel my pain and sorrow and grieve over our loss of Cj. However, I know these moments of pain will become brief as I continue to touch my sorrow and then reflect inwardly. I know the joy that flies to me quickly and washes away my burden. In time, I will listen to Her Music, and it will only bring me joy and beautiful memories.

Thirty-seven

The Wedding

Yesterday's wedding was a very emotional experience for Chuck, Elise and me. It was difficult for me to see the bride walk down the aisle, knowing that Cj would never walk down the aisle with her father. It also brought back memories of Cj and her father walking in front of me down the hospital hallway, arm in arm, with me pushing her I.V. poles. I remember thinking that it looked like Chuck was walking her down the aisle. Now I wonder if he was. Was Chuck walking Cj down the aisle in an early preparation to leave this earth, to leave her parents, to join the Bridegroom on the other side, to join with the Divine? During the ceremony the pastor discussed life with the young couple. He said that there will be times when everything is going so well that others will be envious. Then there will be tragic times. He said these tragic times could actually bring the greatest joy and bring people closer together than they could ever imagine. I remember thinking that this pastor must have made the journey through tragedy.

Tonight I received a telephone call from the groom's father, Charlie. He had not seen me since Cj's memorial service. He sounded unhappy and began telling me that he was concerned about me. He said he had not been able to spend time with me at the wedding and that I looked depressed. Well, my hair was shorter, and I am no longer dyeing it black. Since my hair grayed prematurely, I had been dyeing it black for over fifteen years. Now, many people tell me it is a beautiful white color sprinkled with black. At first, he could not believe that my hair color was natural and thought that I had dyed it gray. I explained that I had stopped dyeing my hair because I wanted to face the unknown of what my hair was like and what it would feel like to be gray. I had faced Cj's illness and the unknown in her passing and received many joyful moments after the tears. To my surprise and joy I have received many compliments on my hair, until tonight. Did I look depressed? I journaled in order to try to gain some insight about this wedding and myself.

041801

I have been thinking about my conversation with Charlie. I don't think I was depressed at the wedding, nor am I depressed now. I think my dear friend was feeling depressed at that moment. I remember hearing the hopelessness in his voice. Charlie told me that he did not know how he would handle the loss of a child. I told him he has been dealing with the loss of a child for many years. Charlie and his wife have had a severely handicapped son for over twenty-five years, and they have been an example to us on how to deal with tragedy. They looked for joy in every set back since their son's infancy, and they never gave up. When it came time to place their son in a setting that provided total care, they could not find a suitable place. They joined with several other families and created a home-based skilled nursing facility for their handicapped children. This home continues to serve their son and handicapped children and families. I realized that they have been our mentors in preparing for Cj's illness and death, and we never knew it.

I shared with Charlie that I believed that there was joy in every tragedy as long as we felt the pain of the loss, mourned it and then looked for the lesson. I am an example of that unique way of dealing with death. I am not depressed. I am not in denial. My heart is joyful and full of love about 85% of the time and I have been healing for only three months. I do feel pain about 15% of the time and my eyes well up with tears, but I am not afraid of that pain nor those tears. I know I feel. By feeling the pain and sorrow I know that I am alive and that I love. I have not closed myself off from life by remaining angry and resentful over the unfairness of it all. If I did then I would be depressed, lacking an interest in anything, being irritable and looking forward to nothing

I celebrate embracing the tough moments that strike. I believe the toughest moments are the death and severe illness of a loved one. However, usually I see a response to loss that is either denial of any pain or anger and resentment that resulted in self-pity and even pity from others. This way blames the tragedy on something (the medical care, the diet, being ignorant as a parent, finances, God, etc.). When we blame it we judge it, fear it and thereby resent it. No growth occurs. The other way is to recognize that life is tragic. We are born and we die, we have and we have not and we get and we lose. Understanding that each loss offers an opportunity for growth brings joy. Over many years I have watched people see tragedy both ways. Mostly, I have watched people take their anger and resentments with them to the grave. What did that contribute to their lives?

Cj's death is the first tragedy in my life, and it is my toughest. No one expects to lose a child. I chose not to remain angry or resentful about our loss. I chose to touch my pain and sorrow, to grieve, to weep, to heal, to find meaning in this tragedy and to grow. I am healing quickly. I do not fit well in a support group, nor any group, where people are still trying to deal with their pain and anger a year or so later. I am not depressed. I love more than I ever did before. I view life differently and feel joyful for what I have. I do not fear anything very long. When a new tough moment happens I know I can feel the pain and sorrow, grieve and mourn, heal, look for the lesson and then joyfully grow. My fears dissolve. I have chosen to wed Joy.

Thirty-eight

Discovery of the Letter

Cj had been gone for three months, and we received a strange letter in the mail. It was addressed to Cj. When we opened it, we discovered that Cj wrote the letter to herself the year before. At first we thought someone had played a thoughtless prank on us. Then we realized that it must have been part of an English assignment. Cj must have written the letter last April, and the teacher collected them. The teacher must have mailed them back to the students this April — one year later.

This letter helped us to see Cj more clearly as a human being. She wrote how she did not like school. She was upset because we were concerned that her report card showed several courses to be incomplete. She was not really happy with life or about being a young teenager. I was amazed that such a letter would come to us just when we were beginning to think of Cj as that "perfect" human being. I wrote to Cj to gain more insight about the letter.

042200

Cj,

You wrote yourself that letter last year. I do not believe in coincidences. I have received some insights about why we received the letter, but I need more information.

Blessed Mom,

The letter was written when I was feeling down. I was different. A lot of the things that made people love me were not easy for me as a human being. Everyone did not love me. We always feel different about humans after they have passed on. I was a teenager. I had my ups and downs. Everyone has ups and downs as part of being on earth. You said several times that I also came to learn things. Why would I be born and not learn anything? What did you learn?

Cj

My angel,

I learned that I can approach my greatest fear, look at it logically and feel the wound, but I cannot heal without experience. My greatest fear was and is loss.

Mom

Beloved Mom,

That is everyone's fear! Loss of anything causes fear, fear of the pain, fear of the unknown and fear of change. We would all love to have things stay the way they are. But, we would crack like a weak tree trunk in the first big gale. Life is facing loss. We begin to face loss as soon as we are born. We lose the comfort of the womb. We lose our mother's breast and then the bottle. We lose the freedom to do what we want and the adult's excitement over our every move. We lose our parents or caretaker because we have to go to school.

We lose the acceptance of our peers as others begin to see differences and develop prejudices. We lose the encouragement to learn and grow at our own pace, and our teachers push us to compete against each other. We begin to lose self esteem as we see others doing better than us, being complimented more, looking better, being thinner, dressing better, having more friends, being more self-assured, having richer parents, and going on better vacations than us. With each loss we feel pain. We begin to lose the dream that life is fair. Someone has something that we don't, and that unfairness becomes painful.

We begin facing a life whereby we are not honored because we are human, but because of our accomplishments. We lose faith that we can do anything even though we may be told that anything is possible. We begin to lose our spark because each time we try to ignite the spark someone manages to inflict pain and the spark goes out. We begin to lose that light that shines and radiates regardless of the situation. We begin to fear the pain that becomes stronger each time we experience a loss. This is the way it is for many of us.

Cj

My child,

If most of us experience pain through loss then who can help us face this pain and fear and the stagnation that it causes? If this is where most of us are, then where lies the help?

Mom,

Help lies in faith and hope. Faith in what, we ask? Faith in something greater than what we know about ourselves. Most of us know only a tiny fraction of ourselves. We only know that part of self that feels fear, anger, happiness, embarrassment, passion, uncertainty, apprehension, etc. We know the part of the self that we see in the mirror everyday and the accompanying judgement we make about our body. We know the part of self we see in our behaviors such as dressing weird, watching TV, studying, going to class, going to work, helping someone less fortunate, avoiding helping someone, going to church, avoiding going to church, voting, not voting, taking medicine, not taking medicine, etc. We often define ourselves by our behaviors, our health and our appearance. When we label and define ourselves, we confine ourselves into a small compartment.

We have difficulty recognizing the part of ourselves that is not and cannot be compartmentalized. This recognition begins to develop when we start to look at our fears. We cannot look at our sorrow or fears unless we feel pain and fear. We must be willing to feel the pain and the fear that comes from loss to get in touch with the more knowledgeable part of ourselves. Unfortunately, we use so many things to avoid feeling the pain and facing the fear. We binge on foods, we smoke, we drink alcohol, we take drugs, we work excessive hours, we watch a lot of TV, we explode at people, we hold onto grudges, we avoid people, we over exercise, we gamble, and we just do and do and do. We do everything, but feel.

The only thing certain in life is loss. We've heard that the only thing certain in life is change. To change something means to lose something. Even if the change is celebrated, something in the old way is remembered and longed for. The greatest awareness of Self comes from feeling sorrow and love. This love is not passion for another human but love for all mankind. The opposite of love and joy is fear and sorrow. We must experience both sides of something to become knowledgeable. We must experience summer and winter to understand the seasons — "For everything there is a season." We must experience fear and sorrow to fully experience love and joy. We must experience sorrow and love to understand feelings. We must understand feelings to begin learning to understand ourselves.

If we want to learn to understand and get in touch with the aspect of ourselves that transcends our body, our emotions, and our intellect, then we must learn to feel. We must be willing to feel the pain from that loss that we previously avoided by using distractions, substances and emotional outbursts. The greatest pain comes from the greatest losses. Pain and sorrow join together to teach us to mourn and experience despair. If we choose to go through this experience with faith and hope that love and joy will follow, then we can ask ourselves what we are learning from the experience. When we can touch the fear we can discover the fear. When we discover the reason for the fear and the specific loss that we fear, then we choose. We can choose to resent that the fear exists and remain fearful or we can use the fear to look for the accompanying joy that follows insight. We can choose to feel the fear, grieve and experience sorrow over the loss. We can cry and begin to heal from a wound that most likely occurred far back in our lives. Then we can experience release from the fear and the pain the wounds created. Release from the fear brings a sense of joy and love of the same magnitude.

Cj

Thank you Cj,

I understand. We have choices in life. We can look at it as unfair and as a struggle. We can look at it as a beautifully designed school where we learn best from our problems. We can blame others for our situations and use avoidances such as drugs, extra work, alcohol, and rage, or we can embrace each situation as an opportunity for growth. We can accept responsibility for our feelings and use them as a wonderful tool for recognizing where we can grow. We can accept fear, pain and sorrow as the most powerful tools for growth. We can grieve, heal and learn. When we understand the lesson, the reward is great joy and love. Then another situation challenges us, and we can face the new challenge with faith and hope that we will learn a new lesson or strengthen a recent one. We can have faith that greater joy and love will follow each new painful experience. We can choose responsibility for our life and embrace each situation as a gift for healing and find greater joy and love than anyone could imagine.

Thank you darling,

Mom

Thirty-nine

Revealing Her Letter

Chuck, Elise and I had not planned to include Cj's letter in *The Healing Room*. The letter was too personal for us to share. The letter showed aspects of Cj that we preferred not to disclose to anyone. We kept it hidden away safely in Cj's cash box. Then a friend read an initial draft of *The Healing Room* a year and a half after we received Cj's letter. She said she wanted to read the letter in order to get to know Cj better. I was still reluctant to include the letter. I took the letter out of the cash box and read it once again.

I had not read her letter for over a year, but this time I began shaking my head in awe. Cj was journaling her own healing room at the age of thirteen. She journaled her pain. I am not sure whether she received any insights after writing, but I am sure she felt better. Her drawing of the bee at the bottom of the letter would make anyone smile. She had drawn a bee and swirling lines indicating its path. Next to it she wrote, "Drunk Bee." I smiled and realized that Cj was still teaching me to face my fears with some humor even though she had been gone over a year. Cj 's letter follows.

April 1999

Things aren't easy. I hope things are easier in one year, which is when I will be reading this letter next. I wish I could go through time to where you (I) am now. I don't know what I am going to do about my report card. I have a lot of friends this year. But unfortunately I am not close to any of them. Maybe when I read this letter I will have some close friends. I love dressing weird and getting second looks. I can't wait until I see RENT. There is not a lot to say. I mean I hope I remember this stuff next year. Elise is going to Outdoor School next week. I am happy for her. The bomb thing was cool. But in a couple of ways I wish it had been a real bomb, and it had gone off. That way I wouldn't have to deal with stuff. But then I think about how it would have affected my family. And I am glad it was just a false alarm. I believe in God and myself and the power of karma. I know I am lucky to have two parents who love me and each other.

I wrote that on Wednesday. What I am about to write I am writing on Friday. Last night I showed my parents my report card. Mom is saying she wants me to repeat 8th grade if my grades don't improve dramatically. Now I wish I was where I am now. I would ask myself so many questions. Mom is talking to me about seeing a shrink. I don't know how I feel about that. I have to get three of my teachers' signatures today to show I asked them about my work. I think I will fake them. But I don't know how I am going to do Mrs. Giles' and Mrs. McEnery's. I know I have to pull myself together if I want to graduate. I know I love Mom and Dad but I want an excuse not to like them. Sometimes I wish I wasn't such a nice person. It would be so much easier. I hear songs every once in a while about how you should enjoy life. Then I think of our society. We are born; we go to school; we get a job; we retire; then we die and that's if you're lucky! There's no real fun in there. I really don't like my life. I wish I were someone else or somewhere else. In someway I can't wait until this life is over. I have no real friends. I mean Elise is great, but I could never tell her any of this stuff. I want so much, but it's like I get so little.

Forty

Labor Pains

I sat with Elise last night and stroked her head. We talked about life and how her experiences will strengthen her as a person after she has healed. We talked about how she must go through her healing in her own way. I was glad she had accepted professional counseling. As we talked, we both began to cry. I held her against me, her head upon my chest. Together, we again felt our pain and sorrow. I rocked Elise and said that we must cry, because tears are a blessing. If we had not loved Cj so much, we would not feel such pain. We both knew that the pain lets us know that our hearts love.

Now it was Good Friday, and Chuck and I had the day off. We were sitting at the table chatting over a cup of coffee. We were talking about Elise and how these times are very difficult for her. She had shared a little about her counseling and said she was experiencing a long-term "adjustment depression" according to the therapist. Our conversation about Elise was painful. I knew that I would gain additional insight if I journaled the conversations I had with both Elise and Chuck.

042101

This morning I talked with Chuck about being with Elise last night. As soon as I mentioned Elise's name my eyes filled with tears, and I was speechless for a moment. Chuck and I looked at each other; we could see the pain in each other's eyes. We sat silently for a while. Then I told Chuck that I was talking to Elise about losing someone early in life. Chuck had lost his dad to heart failure when he was fifteen. I told him I had talked with Elise about his loss and how he had developed such a different view of life at such an early age. For thirty years I've watched how Chuck did not let little things bother him. He has always had a sense of humor about life, and even the difficult times did not hamper his joy of life. At an early age, he had learned what was important — not things, but life. I did not fully understand his intuitiveness until I experienced the loss of Cj.

The Universal Law is the cycle of life and death, of having and losing. This is how it is for everything living on earth. This is how it is for all mankind regardless of gender, race, nationality, religion, etc. We are all born into a body, and that body will die. We all know someone who was born and someone who has died. Through birth we learn to love another; through death we experience loss and learn to touch sorrow and grief. Universal Law also gives us choice. We can choose to be heavily burdened by the sorrow, or we can choose to experience sorrow as waves of pain followed by waves of contentment and even joy.

In looking back over the past three months since Cj's passing, I realize I have been having labor pains. I could fear each pain that hits, tense up, resent its presence, and experience agony. However, I could also recognize each pain as a labor pain knowing that it would not last long. I learned that the pain may last seconds, minutes or even an hour. The pain was the shortest when I did not fear it, when I let myself cry and my heart ache. Then, as suddenly as the wave rolled in, it washed back out. I realized that every time the labor pain subsided, it took some more of my fears with it. Every time I grieved, I feared less, and the burden on my heart became lighter. Every time my heart became lighter, I feared less.

What is the purpose of these labor pains? I think they are for the cycles of Life. They are for Knowledge. We learn and grow by releasing the old. There is fear in releasing the old. The toddler fears releasing the table and taking the first step. At first, the child is afraid of falling and feeling pain. However, after a few bumps, joy follows when crawling gives way to walking. The child learns to walk, run, skate and ride a bike by overcoming the fear of pain. The mastery of each skill brings greater freedom of movement. Joy comes from facing the fear, being willing to feel the pain, and then experiencing the freedom that broadens with each accomplishment. Each step requires labor and pain. Pain gives birth to knowledge and joy when we do not condemn, fear, or blame the pain and sorrow for our predicament.

I have labor pains over Cj's passing. I believe there will always be labor pains from our child's passing. I do not ever expect to get over her death. I will always embrace her life and her death. While alive she taught me so much about how to be a mother and a person. In her death she gave me the opportunity to learn from sorrow. She gave me the opportunity to look at death differently. She gave me the opportunity to reject the temptation of self-pity, resentment, blaming life as being unfair, and the temptation to fear and become hardened against the waves of pain and sorrow. She gave me the opportunity to experience pain and grief in wonderment. I accept these opportunities. I embrace each disappointment, each pain, and each accompanying sorrow as the opportunity to feel, to know that I loved and to gain a greater understanding. I have labor pains. I have them every day. Some are brief and some last longer. I do not fear them. I recognize each wave as a gift. I know that each pain will be accompanied by a new intuitive understanding. I believe this is the way it was meant to be, at least for me.

Forty-one

Popping In

I was driving on an errand thinking peaceful thoughts when all of a sudden Cj popped into my mind. My heart tightened and my throat began to ache. I started to cry. "I miss you so much, Cj," I whispered. I stopped the car and thought of the number of times that Chuck had said that he missed Cj. His statement always concerned me because I did not know for sure how Chuck was dealing with his grief. I only knew how I was dealing with mine. However, whenever he said he missed Cj, suddenly I felt pain and my eyes welled with tears. I reflected for a moment, received some insights and then drove home. As soon as I got home, I pulled out my journal so as not to forget my thoughts.

050200

It is interesting that I always seem to have felt peaceful before Cj popped into Chuck's mind and he made statements about missing her. Sometimes I even felt a little irritated that my peace had been disturbed, but I never mentioned it to Chuck. I just allowed myself to feel the wave of pain.

I reflected on Cj's visit into my thoughts this evening. I do miss her so much and always will. I miss her because I loved being close to her mind, body and spirit for fourteen years. Suddenly, I realized that I feared the pain of missing her too much. I feared that the pain would be less bearable if I missed her even more. Even though I know the pain is the same whether I admit that I miss her or not, I think I have been trying to protect myself from something. If I acknowledge that I loved her physical presence and that I still feel a strong sense of her close beside me, might I have to acknowledge that I fear losing that special sense of closeness? Am I afraid that I will lose all that was Cj?

I recognized that once again fear had crept in and had managed to disguise itself. It kept popping in. Every time Chuck said, "I miss Cj," I became a little irritated because of fear. Well, this evening I touched the fear, and it floated away. I discovered its secret hiding place. I realized that Chuck and I are sharing our grief together. Thoughts about Cj will pop into one of our minds. We will comment on missing her, and this may cause the other a moment of irritation. However, that irritation comes from a fear deep within us. Each time we find fear's hiding place we can touch the fear, let it flutter away and then feel the joy of release.

Forty-two

Happy Birthday, Cj

We had to go to a funeral on Cj's birthday. Chuck's cousin's husband, Art, died at 4:00 a.m. on May 5. During the evening on May 4, there had been a memorial service by the East Bay Cancer Support Group honoring people with cancer and those who have passed away due to cancer. Cj was a special honoree, and I read aloud the poem I wrote, "Once Upon a Lunar Eclipse." Many people had glistening eyes after I read the poem. Then it was interesting to discover that Art passed away from prostate cancer about five hours after that memorial service ended.

Later we found out that the funeral was to be on Cj's birthday, May 10. We had to go because Chuck's parents were away and his sister lives too far away to attend. The funeral service was in Alameda, and then we went to the burial site at St. Mary's Cemetery in Oakland. Amazingly, we found ourselves right back where it all began, near Oakland Kaiser Permanente Hospital and Children's Hospital. We drove past the back of the Chapel of the Chimes Crematorium where Cj was cremated. All of this was coinciding too perfectly to be chance. Besides, I do not believe in chance. That evening, I journaled the experience.

051000

It is amazing that Chuck and I had to spend Cj's birthday at a funeral and then at his cousin's home. This is not at all what we had anticipated we would be doing on her birthday. Elise had gone to the beach with a friend to reflect on Cj. Why would Chuck and I spend this day in such a way? Is there an answer? Then thoughts came to me. Of course there is an answer. Maybe it was just to share the experience and the words that there are no coincidences. Cj was there with us and with the others, as was Art. We did one of the hardest things that we could have possibly done — experience the sorrow of Cj's birthday by going to a funeral and visiting the places where all the sorrow began. We experienced great pain and were surrounded by the pain of others. I think important messages come through many mouths. I know I am often tired and may not always hear the words, but I try to listen to most of them. Maybe I am being tested under stress. It is much easier to listen when there is no stress.

Maybe there were lessons for me to learn, things for me to do and examples that both Chuck and I were setting. Maybe we were brought full circle sooner than we would have chosen. I do listen. I do understand. Maybe Chuck and I were both taking a break from our own personal sorrow to focus our attention on the sorrow of others. Maybe I am learning that stress is only in the mind. I will be where I will be at the time I am supposed to be there. I will do what I will do when it is time for me to do it. This is how it can be if I so choose. I think we are both learning this. It is so much easier than wondering what we are supposed to be doing. It keeps our energy so much higher and allows us to use our minds freely. I think we are both beginning to understand. It is like a carrot on a stick for some. It sounds like nirvana; it is. It is not a place where nothing more is done. Instead, service to mankind becomes the greatest call.

As I continue to follow my intentions, healthier habits are formed. Joy is found. Struggle ceases. All is how it is supposed to be. My mind becomes sharper, but also becomes more humble. I begin to recognize that the answers lie within and that others also have the answers. The messages are all around me.

Happy birthday, Cj. Thank you for your gifts to us today. Thank you for these insights.

Forty-three

Missing You

The past two days have been very difficult. We finally had our Christmas pictures developed and looked at them last night. I was shocked. The last picture we had of Cj was in front of the Christmas tree a week after Thanksgiving. She looked so beautiful with her bright smile and shiny bald head. I looked at it often. Now, I saw her as she was from just before Christmas until her death. I never saw it when I was with her. I don't think I had been allowed to see it. By veiling my eyes I was able to stay very strong and serve Cj up until the very end. Now I saw it in her pictures — impending death. I felt like I experienced Cj's illness and death once again, but this time with no hope. I ached, cried and then wrote Cj a letter.

053000

Hi Cj,

I am really feeling down today. Last night was a difficult evening. Today, I am lamenting and crying, even at work. We finally looked at pictures of you at Christmas time. Your body was giving you pain. We could see that you were dying. We could see it in your eyes and in your complexion. Oh, how my eyes were veiled. I miss you. I am worried about Elise.

She misses you. Sometimes I am so tired of the pain. Do you have a message for me?

Hi Mom,

You heard the words from your friend. Remember that messages are all around. The first year is the most difficult, the second easier. You have to go through this. You can avoid agony and anguish, but you cannot heal if you avoid the pain. Every time you feel pain you discover something. It is okay to cry anywhere. There is a time and place to cry, but you may not be sure where that time or place is.

Of course you miss me. You love me. However, at first you had only developed the ability to love me as a tangible being. On earth, old programs, parental worries, and society's expectations get in the way of total love. When a loved one passes away the old programs quickly go away. You no longer get upset that I do not do the dishes, leave the attic a mess, forget to flush the toilet, don't do my homework, get short with you, etc. All these thoughts (mental plays) interfere with the ability to feel the pure light of love. You were busy being my parent and trying to help me evolve into a successful member of society according to society's definitions.

You are no different than any other parent. Shaping children is one of the parent's roles. However, you learned that you really did not have control over me even before I got sick. No one has control over another human being. You tried to learn from the tragic experience that was given to you. You are learning everyday. But, learning also takes time. The whole lesson cannot be learned in a month. It will take you a lifetime. You might think you understand, but to integrate this experience into your mind, body, emotions and spirit will take time. You are having a human experience. You are going through great pain, one of the greatest pains that some-one can experience.

Yes, you understand that some people go through greater tragic experiences. Every tragic experience has a purpose. Yours is to continue to try to learn to be in the moment. If you feel sad, feel sad. If you feel joy, feel joy. Do not judge yourself. Do not feel that you need to be stronger than anyone else.

You ask me where I am? You know. You have intuition. You have been busy lately and that is fine. I am right beside you. I am not sleeping. I am not sleeping on this side. I do not need to sleep. I am wherever you think I am on the earth plane. You just can't see the me you knew. You wouldn't want to. You are blessed to be on the earth plane. A big lesson for mankind is that people are born and they die; they begin class and they graduate. You are in school. You never really liked school, and your schoolmates slowly moved away to another world. The difference is that I did not leave, I transformed. When you feel me you are joyful. However, it is very difficult being on the earth plane and being intuitive at all times. It takes practice. Yes, it is possible.

There is no "way" to do anything except that way which feels best. You know what you want. Anyone can have what you want. You want what you want because you believe. Have patience. You miss me because you love.

Cj

Forty-four

Writing That Letter

I knew that writing letters to people who did not know about Cj's illness and passing would be one of the hardest things I had to do. I procrastinated writing this letter for six months, and I cried while my fingers fumbled over the keyboard. I cried and lamented when I read it. Chuck cried aloud when he read it. It still causes us pain and sorrow when we read it over. Therefore, I knew that we were not yet ready to return to this vacation spot. However, I knew that the people who read it would have had the opportunity to mourn and then accept Cj's passing. They would be prepared for her absence when we return. Anyone who has experienced loss will have a letter to write. If we heal each time we return to a painful experience and grieve and mourn, then writing the letter was a healing experience.

June 23, 2000

Dear Sandy and Ellie and R-Ranch Partners;

It is with great sadness that we send you this news. We apologize for the delay, but this has been the most difficult letter to write. Our daughter, Cj Bohntinsky, passed away on January 20, 2000. She was suddenly diagnosed in September 1999, with a rare form of leukemia (called myelodysplastic syndrome). Her bone marrow suddenly quit making blood. This happened after her first week of high school as a freshman, so we're blessed to have a freshman picture. She underwent two rounds of chemotherapy and was doing well until a wisdom tooth came in after Thanksgiving. This resulted in a sinus infection. Cj had no immune system as she had no white blood cells. Dori was Cj's match as a bone marrow donor, but Cj passed away before the bone marrow transplant could ever be initiated.

Cj was an inspiration to all (family, friends and the medical field) during her battle. We tried to approach each challenge as an opportunity to learn and grow. We feel very blessed that Cj went on a ventilator and was sedated into sleep five days prior to her death. She had developed pneumonia, and the doctors told her that they would wake her when her lungs were better. However, the infection only got worse. Cj never knew that she was going to pass away but instead continued to put the medical profession in awe by asking about the ventilator procedure, the medications to be used, the side effects, and what they were going to do if she began to bleed. After the doctors answered her questions to her satisfaction, she gave them her permission. She left this world having touched the hearts and having taught many.

One doctor asked us to share with others how we had managed Cj's illness and finally made the decision to let her pass away. We have created a foundation, called the CJ Foundation. Dori is also writing a book about our experience, how we allowed ourselves to feel the pain and experience the grief of every disappointment. Each time we touched a sorrow we later discovered a gift of joy. The book is called *The Healing Room.*

Cj loved R-Ranch. She started going there when she was one-year old. She learned to walk, swim, ride horses, fish (she caught a turtle once), dance, ride a bike, play Pinochle and Cribbage at the Ranch. We have many wonderful pictures of her growing up at the Ranch and many treasured memories. The Ranch is going to be the most difficult place to return to. It causes great pain just to write this letter. We are no longer that family of four reading books or playing cards near the pool or beside the recreation room. We will be back when it is time, because we know that the Ranch will be a healing place for us.

Sincerely,
Chuck, Dori and Elise Bohntinsky

Forty-five

The Vacation

We went on a vacation up to Victoria, British Columbia in August. I don't think that we would have gone on vacation in 2000 if it had not been for my cousin who insisted that we come for a visit to their home. I knew that it would be difficult to face the first vacation without Cj. However, the few days prior to the vacation were uneventful. I was focusing on the things that needed to be completed at work before leaving. The night before our trip was spent packing, and I noticed that I was being a little short with Elise. But, I had always been a little nervous the evening before leaving for vacation, so I did not give it much thought.

The next morning, Chuck, Elise and I were packing the car. There was no suitcase for Cj in the trunk. Her sleeping bag was not in the back seat. There sitting on her side was her favorite stuffed dog, a gift Elise had given her while she was in the hospital. I went and sat down in the kitchen and cried. I felt the pain of Cj's absence. This is why I was irritable last night and this morning. I missed Cj. My tension had not been so much about me, but rather apprehension about having to feel the pain from loss once again. I felt the pain, cried and then thought, "Now I am ready for our trip."

We made it up to Victoria without too many difficult moments. I made a journal entry about the trip the next day, but left the entry incomplete. I did not finish the entry until I returned home from our vacation.

081500

Chuck, Elise and I drove up north for the first time since Cj passed away, and this was our first vacation as a family of three. The first couple of hours were relaxing. We had driven this same route a few months ago, so I did not have any "Cj Firsts." As we headed farther up north, we began seeing the familiar landscape and towns that we had driven past for fourteen years on our way to R-Ranch where we spent many weekends and vacations. We had decided earlier that we would not return to the ranch for at least a year. It would be one of the most difficult experiences for us to face because so many of our memories of Cj growing up are from the ranch. It was there that she learned to swim, ride a bike, ride a horse, dance and just relax. That is the place where we learned to relax and learned to play together as a family. Now we were getting closer and closer to Red Bluff and the turn off to the ranch. I felt tears begin to flow down my cheeks. I wiped at my eyes as we drove on. We were not ready to face the ranch, but here we were driving past the turn off that was only forty-five minutes from the place that holds so many memories. I shook my head. My heart hurt, my throat tightened and the tears kept falling. We all checked in with each other and asked if everything was OK. We all admitted that the journey was becoming painful, but we knew that the pain would decrease as long as we continued to reflect on our feelings.

We continued up north and approached Mt. Shasta. We talked about how we had visited the mountain only a few years earlier and had taken a tour of the caverns. I thought about Cj sitting by me on the boat while crossing the lake, riding on the old creaky bus and walking through the caves. I shook my head as I silently wept and thought, "Never again with Cj."

As we traveled north the landscape became less familiar. We had only traveled this way a couple of times, so the pain from the reminders of places we had visited began to subside. We had faced the worst part of this trip: the memories of places we had often been together. I sighed. We all sighed. As we traveled on we became more aware of the beautiful scenery. We looked for the place in Oregon where we had stopped and had a picnic when Cj was only eight years old. When we finally recognized the turnoff we said, "That had been a great picnic." I noted that there was no pain and no tears. I felt peaceful.

All of a sudden I began to smile. Once again we had managed. I knew that we would not only be okay, but we would actually enjoy this vacation. I knew that we would have moments of sadness because Cj was not there with us. That was true. We missed her throughout the trip. However, I knew that she was in a better place. I knew that we needed the vacation to help us experience some joy and happiness by seeing the beauty of nature and being with loved ones.

I did not need to make any additional journal entries during the trip. I had already felt my pain and understood. "That had been a great picnic." In many ways life with Cj seemed like a picnic. Problems and issues had already disappeared. We had begun to equate our happiness with Cj being with us. It seemed that without Cj, life was not the same; therefore, Cj must have been responsible for our happiness. We all knew that this was not true, but it is very easy for our minds to begin to believe this. I knew that life had not always been happy when Cj was with us. We had faced the same challenges of most families. Cj had not made us happy. Cj was part of our happiness as a family. A segment of that happiness was now missing.

I began to understand that we would eventually be happy again. I began to look forward to the vacation. I looked forward to experiencing some fun and being happy. I would begin creating new memories. I knew that the new memories would be mixed with the sorrow of missing Cj during this vacation. However, I knew that each sad moment would be accompanied by a moment of equivalent joy.

Forty-six

Why?

I find myself asking, "Why?" Why did she get sick? Why was it such a hopeless illness? Why did she have to die so young? Why did she have to have pain in the end? Why was she taken from us? Why were we the parents to experience this loss of a beloved child? Why did Elise have to be the one to suffer the loss of her sister? Why are we the ones that have to live with each other's sorrow? Why did she leave us? The question " Why?" could go on and on. Then, I was listening to a song today and caught the short refrain, "Ask not why." Interestingly, I thought, "Why?" Then, I wrote.

090100

Is asking, "Why?" like the child that keeps asking the parent a question until the question cannot really be answered? What keeps the earth warm? The sun heats the earth. How does the sun heat the earth? By its energy. Why does it give off energy to the earth? Hmm.

I thought about how once we reach a certain age we know that with life comes death. No one is immune from experiencing the loss of a loved one if they have loved. Since Cj passed away, I have heard of others going through sorrow. More children are being or have been diagnosed with the same illness as Cj. A young colleague lost his best friend to cancer. A young mother lost her forty two-year-old husband to a brain tumor. A friend lost her elderly mother, and my parents' friend lost his wife suddenly to bone cancer. I am not isolated. I am not alone. I am just not one of those who have not mourned death yet. However, I do not know what hidden sorrows others may be experiencing. Many have lost loved ones to drugs, crime, bitter arguments, lack of acceptance, lack of forgiveness, etc. I have received support from my family, friends and co-workers during my period of healing because they know about my suffering. Do those with hidden sorrows receive any comfort at all?

When I ask, "Why?" I am questioning the way of the Universe. Even stars die. Asking why does not help me heal; it makes me feel like I am a victim. I do not choose to be a victim. Every time I ask why, my heart sinks. Maybe when I ask why, Cj has to come to me and hold up my sinking heart. If there are no available answers to the "why's" then Cj has to do a lot of work to comfort me. When I lovingly think, "It is what it is," my heart lightens. I do not love Cj any less because I accept. Maybe I have even learned to love her more. I am learning to release her. I am learning to let her fly free. When I "let it be," I am loving, creative, and empathetic to the suffering and joy of all mankind. When I love, I am joyful. When I ask, "Why?" I feel sorrow. Maybe that is the lesson.

Forty-seven

When It's Time to Grow Up...
(By Elise)

Elise had to write a college-entrance essay when she was a senior in high school. In many ways, I felt this essay was a gift to me. It was part of Elise's healing room. Though we had not discussed it, I learned that Cj had helped Elise develop one of the most important aspects of humanity — compassion. I felt great joy and humble pride.

092000

For a large portion of my life I had believed that the only way for me to stand out in life was to be smart. I was always striving to earn the highest grade in the class, to set all the curves and to win the most prestigious awards. I believed that the only thing that set me apart from others was my intelligence, and I wanted to be remembered for it. As a result, I hid many parts of my true self. The carefree, humorous, and creative sides of me were hidden in the fear that they would be made fun of. I was too afraid that I would appear to be stupid. So instead I became what I thought others wanted me to be. I continued on this path of naiveté until my world was turned upside-down and my journey of self-discovery began.

My younger sister, Cj, and I were exact opposites from the day she was born. She was the creative child, always causing trouble. Cj loved to color on the walls, take apart my toys, and fill all the soap dispensers at home with red dye. As we got older she was the one who stood out in the world. Her unique style, sparkling personality, and amazing ability to love unconditionally made a lasting impression on everyone she met. I was praised for my intelligence, but Cj was praised simply because she had learned to truly accept herself.

In September of my junior year, Cj was diagnosed with a rare disease called Myelodysplastic Syndrome. Her body stopped making blood, resulting immediately in a hospital room and strong doses of chemotherapy. I watched her suffer for four months, yet she never gave up her positive outlook on life and never failed to smile. All the nurses and doctors loved her, aware of the special person that they had in their care. It amazed me that she continued to touch the lives of every person she met. On January 20, 2000, my life changed drastically, as did the person I wanted to be. Every meaningful journey has to begin with a tragedy, mine was no different, and it began with the death of my sister.

I had always heard that after someone you love dies you go through five steps of mourning: denial, anger, bargaining, depression, and finally acceptance. After Cj was first diagnosed, I wouldn't let myself believe that there was even a possibility of her dying. I was sure that we were going to grow old together and that I would always have her to hug. It wasn't until two days before her death that I accepted the possibility of her death. When she died, I became angry that someone so special had to die so young. It seemed so cruel and unnecessary. I didn't understand why she had to die, and I couldn't find an explanation. I was mad at the world. Even though I refused to believe in the chance that Cj might die, I did experience bargaining. I vowed that if she got better we would do everything together, that she could always hang out with my friends and go anywhere with me. Cj considered me to be her best friend, and I was determined to act like it. Depression began to play a large part in my life a few months after Cj died. Every afternoon I would come home from school, curl up in a quilt and either sleep or stare blankly at a wall. I couldn't find motivation to do anything; my heart hurt too much. I could only focus on memories that were continuously floating through my head: Cj watching Saturday morning cartoons, Cj baking some mystery dessert, and the two of us sitting and talking to each other about everything. Finally I got frustrated and forced myself to get moving again. I think that by remembering all the good times we shared I was finally able to accept Cj's death as being the best possible thing for her. If she had survived, her life would have been filled with perpetual pain and more suffering; this would have been too difficult for everyone. Instead, with her death she continued to teach lessons to others. I began to reflect on my entire life, both in relation to her and in relation to the world. I realized for the first time that I had been living a superficial life caring mainly for my own happiness. It was time for a change.

Looking back at my life now, I see some very drastic changes. I have finally learned to accept myself, not just my intelligence but everything. No longer do I mold myself to society, but rather I do whatever I feel comfortable doing and makes me the happiest. By casting off society's shell of fashion and popular outfits, I've developed my own personal style. My confidence in myself has grown at an astounding rate. Instead of waiting to be asked my opinion or hiding timidly in the corner, I have learned to freely express my opinions and stand up for myself. The sides of my personality that I have hidden for so long are now apparent. I can play the group jester, no longer fearing that I will appear childish. I try to live life to the fullest and remain cheerful, enjoying and learning from every experience. My sister's ability to completely love others is beginning to show through me as I begin to completely love myself. Friendships have become stronger and more meaningful. By learning to accept myself I've learned to completely accept my friends; I can recognize the qualities that make them so special. My intelligence is still very important to me, but not for the same reasons. I now strive for good grades because I want to; I love the challenge and the rewarding feeling I get after accomplishing something. I may still be remembered for my intelligence, but it is no longer crucial. I'd rather be remembered for the person that I have become. I think that I have finally grown up. I know that I am ready to try anything and will be able to survive.

The changes in my life have had only one set back. I grew up too fast, never getting to fully enjoy my teenage years. I no longer fit into the high school atmosphere; I am out of place there. School is not much of a challenge to me, and the people are often hard to understand. My ears do not perk up to the gossip of who is dating whom, and who is driving what car. I'd rather discuss more worldly issues with people of a similar mindset. I feel that I have learned everything that I can from high school; it is time for me to take another step in my journey. In January, I will take that step and graduate from high school early. I'm not trying to escape from an uncomfortable situation; I'm simply beginning a search for new experiences that will help me to develop even further as an individual.

I have been prepared for the world by tragedy. Cj taught me more with her death than I could have ever learned on my own. Through her example I hope to touch many lives and share the gift of love that she has left me. I like to think that Cj lives on in me and that in a sense, we will grow old together.

Forty-eight

Decorating Again

One of Cj's favorite holidays was Halloween. We have had a Halloween party every year since before she was born. She grew up around the decorations, which included flying bats, hanging skeletons, witches, mummies, Draculas, pumpkins, etc. Every year new decorations were added. Every year our old friends came and then their children. Then our children invited their friends. The Halloween party became an annual tradition, but I did not realize its importance until last year when Cj was sick. She wanted the house decorated for Halloween. She wanted a party. She was in the hospital getting chemotherapy, and she had no immune system. A party was not possible.

Last year we did not feel comfortable decorating the house with goblins when we were praying so hard for her recovery, nor was there time. Cj agreed to forego having the house decorated for Halloween if we completely decorated for Christmas (all three artificial trees and the Christmas village included). We also compromised by decorating her hospital room with Halloween decorations. We had decorated her room every time she went to the hospital. In fact we were surprised to find out that we were the only family that the nurses had ever seen decorate a hospital room. Cj loved the decorations. The gaiety of the room delighted her visitors, and the nurses often took their breaks in Cj's room.

A year had passed since that partyless Halloween. Chuck and I decided that we had to keep on with the tradition of the Halloween party. Elise and her friends were looking forward to it. I did not realize that I would experience such pain from decorating.

102100

We took out the boxes of decorations early in October. I always began decorating the first of October because we had accumulated years of decorations. However, this time the boxes remained piled up on the garage floor. I was busy doing other things and had no time to start decorating. The weeks passed by. Now I had one week left, and I had to start. I opened up the boxes and began putting up the characters, setting out the dummies, and blowing up the skeletons. It seemed like any other preparation for the party.

As I went through the pile of paper decorations, I started finding the very old ones. Cj and Elise used to laugh about the certain posters that "scared" them when they were little girls. Cj was not here to laugh nor to help me put up decorations. I found the funny pumpkin Cj had made when she was in first grade. I taped it to her door. As I stared at it I felt such emptiness. I wiped the tears from my cheeks, took a deep breath and went back to the pile of decorations. I put another one up. I found several decorations that Elise made in grade school and put them up next to her door. I went back to the pile of decorations, stared at them and then at Chuck who was sitting on the couch. "This is really hard," I whispered.

I went off and cried. I cried more than I had in a couple of months. I ached once again. I missed Cj so much. I wanted her back. I wanted to hear her begging me to make her a new outrageous costume. I wanted her in my arms. I wanted to hear her laugh. My tears took a long time to stop. I cried as I wrote about my pain. Then, my tears stopped, and the pain eased up. I knew from months of experience that I had choices. I could continue to focus on Cj's absence, feel sorry for myself and possibly even become bitter. I could continue to feel the pain that way. My other choice was to breathe deeply and reflect on the experience. Meaning could come as I continued writing. I had learned that the lesson would come if I trusted reflection.

I reflected on the pain and grief that I had just experienced. For me the lesson was nothing at all like I expected. I lost my mother last month on September 13. She passed away eight months after Cj's death. My mother was able to remain at home, and I had focused on the joy I felt that she died peacefully. I had been able to help tend to her and felt honored to have served her during the final week of her life. I knew she was no longer in discomfort. My concerns had turned to my father. Also, I did not want the people at my work to be overly concerned about me. I said, "I am doing well."

I was not doing well. I had noted that I was taking on more and more tasks and keeping very busy. My time was being filled with all kinds of things, and they were all justifiably important. I figured this was just how things were going to be for a while. I had been telling myself, "I don't have time to start on the decorations." But, that was not really true. The truth was that I was not making time to mourn her death. I was avoiding mourning. I was avoiding grief. I did not want to go through it again so soon. I fooled myself into thinking that I did not need to mourn because my mother's passing had been different. The result was that my life was becoming full of "things to do" and I was feeling greater dissatisfaction each day. I took on additional obligations and tasks to ease my dissatisfaction. I was really adding tasks to avoid mourning.

Well, tonight I mourned. I thought it was for Cj. Maybe it was. Now I realize that it was also for my mother. Maybe I will mourn them both together as they are hard to separate; mother and daughter. What is important is that I mourned. I felt the pain and stayed with it. I grieved, even though my understanding was limited. By doing so I released something that had been building unnoticed for a month. Now, I feel more at peace. I feel ready to face the pile of decorations. However, it is late, so I will decorate tomorrow.

Forty-nine

The Grinch

Chuck and I saw a movie during the holiday season. The movie made me think about the similarities between the main character and what Chuck and I were going through. I decided to write a Christmas letter, because I knew many would want to know how we were managing our losses. I called the Christmas letter *The Grinch.*

11/27/00

Dear friends and family;

We wish you a very peaceful and loving holiday season. This is a page from *The Healing Room,* and we would like to share it with you during this season.

Chuck and I have just seen the movie *The Grinch Who Stole Christmas.* We both missed Cj. She would have loved the children's laughter during the movie. While watching the show, I imagined her letting out belly laugh after belly laugh because I was even giggling. Families sent out ripples of joyous energy as they began the celebration of the holiday season. I felt such tenderness towards the parents and children. I wondered whether someone else in this theater might be going through sorrow from the loss of a loved one.

As we walked out of the theater, my heart became heavier and heavier with each step. No longer was I being carried along on the magic carpet of fantasy as people went their separate ways. On the way home I saw the first colorful lights of the season and my body ached. The holiday season is not the gifts; it is the families being together. That was one of the messages of the movie. I thought, "Our family is not together. Both Cj and Mom have left us this year." I ached with sorrow.

I know that so many things will be reminding us of Cj's absence, and I am not sure what to do. Do I hang her stocking? Do I put her name on the sugar cookies? Do I even bake sugar cookies? Do we hang her personal ornaments on the tree? At least we don't have to wonder about putting up the Dickens Village. Cj loved putting up the village, and we knew last January that we would not be able to face it. We were not able to take it down, so we just left it up in the bay window all year. We only have to decide when to light it.

I reflected on the movie. The Grinch felt such pain in his heart as it began to grow. At first, I thought the Grinch was having a heart attack as he writhed on the ground clutching his pounding heart. Then he said, "I feel, and I am leaking," as the tears rolled down his cheeks. What an ache, especially this time of year. I could avoid the decorating and avoid the ache and pain in my heart that each traditional item will trigger. But then, I could become like The Grinch whose heart shrunk each time he avoided his pain. That was when he refused to feel, became bitter and ostracized himself from the world. No, when The Grinch finally touched his pain he found love. So, I will continue to follow, maintain and help in our family traditions even though my heart pounds and hurts often during this holiday season.

This was Cj's most favorite time of the year. I will hurt for her presence. But each time I hurt I will remember her smile, laughter and kindness. I will hurt like The Grinch. I feel my heart's pain and my eyes "leak." I feel the pain of the loss of our child, and therefore, I feel the pain of mankind. I will not become bitter but instead choose to grow in my ability to love. This season I will find and understand peace on earth and feel good will towards all men.

Fifty

A Family Matter

The gatherings with our extended family have had an undercurrent since Cj's passing. We are very close to our parents and siblings, but in the past did not spend every holiday with them. Now we have been gathering with the extended family instead of continuing on with the traditions we built around the four of us. We abandoned our own celebration of Easter and the 4th of July this year. Chuck and I could not bear the pain of the reminder that we were a threesome. So, we joined our family in these celebrations. We celebrated when we did not feel like celebrating.

My mother assured that we all gathered together for birthdays, Thanksgiving and Christmas. Mom and Cj are not here with us now, but we have been striving to keep the traditions the same. We have been acting joyful around each other when maybe we are all really crying inside. However, even our internal tears did not always seem to mix well with the celebrations. Finally, a family situation occurred which resulted in a misunderstanding and pain. I knew that even this experience would provide me with a lesson if I journaled.

12200

I allowed my December birthday to be celebrated by the whole family due to their urging. I had really wanted to celebrate it alone with Elise and Chuck. I was actually distracted all day by activities, and I thought I was happy. I actually thought, "I am proud of myself that I did not get depressed on my birthday." I made it through that day without feeling sorrow.

I still felt happy on Monday, the following morning. I continued to feel proud that I had gotten through my birthday without Cj or my mom there, and I appreciated how caring everyone had been. By mid-morning, I received a telephone call at work. My world fell apart. One of my sisters called to tell me that I had said the wrong words regarding my birthday present and about food for Christmas. I thought she was calling to tell me how well the party went, and I was just about to thank her for all the work she did to make my birthday special. Instead, I went into shock. The pain hit hard, and I became very angry. I felt she was venting and releasing her disappointment by putting the burden on me even though I was at work. My voice cracked. I know I yelled and then hung up. I sat there numb. We all knew better than to treat each other this way. What happened?

It got worse. I remained silent. My sister expressed herself on the message machines. She made her boundaries clear; several areas being ones that I held dear. I felt like I had been kicked down when I was just getting to my knees. I felt it would be best to just let things cool down. However, it ended up that things cooled down too much, and we were not all together for Christmas; my sister did not come. Once again I felt loss, pain and sorrow. I felt angry and unsettled for over a week. I wondered why this had happened. What had I done to deserve more pain? I had only been trying to do what everyone wanted. I had celebrated, even when I felt like being alone and crying.

I continued to feel sad and was preoccupied by the situation. How could this event cause me pain when I had just been through eleven months of dealing with Cj's death and three months dealing with my mother's? It seemed to be so trivial in comparison. It took me awhile before I could let it go and reflect on the lesson. My lesson would not become clear until I touched and then let go of my feelings.

I had thought I was doing a good job in healing from my losses. I continued to go to work and take care of my family after losing Cj. I helped my mother during her illness. I helped my father after my mother's death. I remained strong. I dried my tears quickly when I was in public. I lamented in private. I continued to write this book to share with others how writing helped in my healing.

I did what I was "supposed to do." I went to work when I did not want to work. I smiled when I wanted to cry. I shared words of encouragement when I wanted to say, "I hurt, and I want Cj back." I allowed myself to be surrounded by others when I just wanted to be alone. I celebrated with the family when I did not want to celebrate. Did I ever do what I wanted to do? I can't remember, and I am not sure.

Why did my sister get so angry with me? I will never know. I am not even sure why I got angry with her. Maybe I expected special treatment. Maybe I expected a reward for my suffering and good behavior. Instead, I was finally pushed until I broke. The veil of my illusion tore. I had not gotten angry. I couldn't get angry with Cj. It was not her fault she had gotten so sick. I could not get angry with my mother, for it was not her fault that her heart failed. I had done everything possible in trying to heal, so how could I get angry with myself?

I had read that one of the steps of mourning is anger. I did not agree, as I had not gotten angry over the loss. I seemed to be healing rapidly. Even my therapist said so. I knew that I had been healing. Only something was missing. The feeling of anger was missing. Anger is different from bitterness. My anger was a brief explosion. Bitterness lasts much longer. My anger helped me reflect on myself in a different way. Before I had been focusing on the pain and sorrow from my loss. My anger helped me to focus on myself.

I am going to start learning to do what I want to do. I had expected a reward for my good behavior. There is no reward. I am going to learn to reward myself. No, I am not going to abandon my life and live on a tropical island. I am just going to learn to live. I am learning to feel more than just pain. I am learning to focus on different feelings now. At times, I dare say, I have even felt bliss.

My pain in losing Cj is not greater than the rest of the family's. It is only different. It is because my family also felt love and pain that we could become angry. Now I honor that anger which at first seemed so unnatural. After eleven months of pain, it was the anger that finally shattered the veil of my defenses and helped me see myself.

Fifty-one

Closure with Family

One of my sisters and I had not spoken since the day after my birthday when I hung up the telephone on her. She sent me a letter about two weeks after my outburst wondering why she had not received an apology. I had not contacted her because certain things that she said on my message machine made me think it would be best if we both reflected on the issues. I had hoped that she would look at both points of view and then just let go of it. However, her letter made me realize that I needed to write to her. Not only did my letter let her know my feelings, it also provided me with more insight into myself. We were then able to celebrate my mother's birthday in February comfortably and lovingly as a whole family.

010201

Dearest Sister,

Thank you for your letter. It made me realize that closure was needed. I had hoped that you might have slowly seen the situation from both of our points of view, no one right and no one wrong. I was called at work on a Monday morning to be vented on. I was exhausted from three solid weeks of serving people. I had not wanted to celebrate my birthday. I did not want to go to work on Monday, but I had to because someone else was off. Like many other days, I cried in the bathroom and then shook my head and headed off to work.

I had just told two staff members that I had not gotten depressed on my birthday for the first time that I could remember. I made it through my first birthday without my daughter there and had told Chuck and Elise that I was proud that I had not gotten depressed. I later realized that pride certainly comes before a fall, because part of my world fell apart that Monday. First, I was given good news, then bad news about what I said regarding my present (for which I apologized) and then bad news again about another statement I had made. I lost my temper. It was "the straw that broke the camel's back." It angered me to receive this information on Monday morning at work in order to lighten your burden. I felt like I had been kicked back down when all year I had been trying to at least get back up to my knees.

I did not condone my behavior, nor did I condone yours. I did not feel it was time to call you. I came home to more messages. These hit me in the places that were very dear, and Elise came home finding me in tears. I did not believe you wanted to talk since all communication was by messages left while I was at work.

I do not feel that an apology is necessary, except maybe to say that I am sorry that I stepped on your feet during the dance of life. We stepped on each other's. We both probably feel that we were tripped and then kicked. However, for me that is what life is about. People will push my buttons, I will step back and lick my wounds and then reflect on my lesson. I learned and grew a lot from all of this. I saw no need to defend myself. That is all I can tell you. I live in a different world.

I harbor neither anger nor any regrets. I had to release these concepts over the past year, or I would not have remained sane. Now I try to use life to love, serve and to grow from my lessons. That does not mean that I do not push buttons or get mine pushed. I just use them to grow. When I am done serving and growing I will go home. I have sent you only love over the past couple of weeks. I can give you nothing more.

We all swim in different oceans. Neither of us can understand those oceans. I know your boundaries now and I think you know mine. I have no expectations of myself; I live moment by moment. I have no expectations of anyone. I have new life situations to deal with. This one is gone, released and I feel only love and joy.

Thank you for the Christmas gifts; they contain a lot of love. I look forward to seeing you and celebrating Mom's birthday on February 17.

Love,
Dori

Fifty-two

The Anniversary

I had thought about the anniversary of Cj's passing for a couple of months. Elise, Chuck and I had decided to be together. I was not sure what we were going to do that day and certainly not sure how we would feel. I did know that it was important that we go somewhere. I selected a place to go for the weekend where Cj had never been. This way we could focus on ourselves as a family of three instead of feeling nostalgic regarding a place that we had visited with Cj. I wanted my thoughts about Cj to be about her, not about a place where she had been.

012001

Today is the anniversary of Cj's passing. We did not know what to expect. The three of us decided to go somewhere different and spend the night. We went to a place on the coast where Cj had never been. We found an old motel right on the water with waves breaking onto the sea wall that protected the parking lot. There were two knolls, one on the right and the other on the left.

We collected driftwood and rocks for the garden during the afternoon. Just before sundown we climbed to the top of the knoll on the left and watched the sun set into the ocean. We mentioned how no sunset would ever be like this one because all sunsets are different. The clouds will be a little different, the air a little different, the water different, and therefore, the sunset a little different. We missed Cj. We all miss her differently because each of our lives with her was different. Like a sunset, there will be no other Cj.

We went out for dinner. We could see the waves from our table, and I imagined Cj out there playing in the waves. She will never be cold. We ate a meal in celebration of Cj's enjoyment of eating. She will never be hungry or have to eat vegetables. We had dessert in memory of Cj's love of sweets. She will never have another cavity or gain another pound. We listened to the band playing music. She will never have to turn her music down or worry that she does not have batteries for her CD player. I felt that she was content and happy.

In the morning we walked on the beach and collected rocks. Strangely, during the night a wide variety of rocks, large and small, arrived on the beach. We also noticed that they had disappeared from the spot where we were collecting them the day before. We slowly began collecting the green ones, then red ones, and then the beige. As we collected the rocks, the waves kept coming closer and closer onto the beach. I began noticing that the waves were taking the rocks away. Even the large ones were disappearing. The waves that had brought the rocks during the night were now taking them back into the ocean.

I was a little sad to see the rocks go. I enjoyed their beauty against the sand, but I also marveled at how one wave could take back so many. I also knew that the rocks were not far away, just hidden from my view. They would return when the ocean was ready to scatter them back onto the beach.

I thought about how similar these rocks were to life. Life comes into being on the tide of love's joining. Love brings life into view of mankind. We celebrate and collect these lives to create our families. When it is time, the tides of Love take the lives back and gather them away from our view. These lives are still there; we just can't see them. This is how I am learning to think of Cj. She is still here. She is just out of my view. I can sense her and feel her love.

The tides of Love will bring in more lives. I will always cherish and celebrate these lives. I love my life more than ever before. In time, the tides will come in and gather more of my loved ones from my view. That will be all right. I have been through two of the cycles now — my daughter and my mother — and have no fear of the sadness. I have survived my pain. I have grown from my sorrow. I faced one of mankind's greatest fears, the loss of a child, and I am still here. My insights have even provided me with glimpses of bliss.

Maybe this is what life is all about. As soon as we arrive it is only natural that we begin to return. We just don't know when or who will go first. Maybe the gift for experiencing such sorrow from loss is that death no longer holds fear. I no longer fear death. My father says he no longer fears death. Maybe, when we no longer fear death, we no longer fear. Maybe it is when we are released from fear that the Healing actually begins.

It has been a year since Cj passed away. I have been in the Healing Room for a year. I still cry. I still miss her. I love her. I feel her. I feel joy. I have very little fear. I feel. I am alive. I love. I am growing. I am continuing to heal. Maybe when all my healing is complete, I will leave the Healing Room and be taken back by the tides. I will join Cj and the others that were gathered back into the ocean of the Universe before me.

Fifty-three

And Then There Were Three

I was sitting on the couch reading a book about how it takes time to heal and how the healing period after injury is the gestation of wisdom. I began to sob. How long is that healing period especially when injuries seem to be piling up? It was the day before my father's funeral. He died March 11, two days short of six months after my mother's death. In one day, he went from being a healthy eighty-four-year-old man who was helping others in the community to a bed-ridden patient hospitalized with congestive heart failure and pneumonia. In just nine days he was gone. He is now with Cj and my mother. The day before my father's funeral, I cried and asked, "Who am I mourning?" The words came to me, "And then there were three."

I was mourning all three: Cj, my mother and my father. The familiar feeling of tightness in my chest had returned. I was sobbing and tears were dampening my cheeks. I ached for the faces and voices of three very dear people. I wondered what I could do to experience this sorrow while at the same time ease my pain? That quiet voice within said, "Go write."

031801

When my father died I was somewhat hesitant to call my friends. I felt an emotion that held no word. In a year and a half my friends received multiple sad messages from us. The first messages began with the diagnosis of Cj's illness, her slow declines mixed with our hope for recovery, her passing, my mother's decline, and then my mother's passing. Now I needed to inform them about my father's death. I don't think that I felt embarrassed, but I felt conspicuous. Was there something wrong with me that I was experiencing so much tragedy over eighteen months? After receiving the news of my father's illness and death, a friend hugged me and tried to console me by saying, "Now it is over, things happen in threes."

I do not understand why people are more relieved after three things have happened. It is a very common saying that "things happen in threes." Now during another great moment of sorrow, the gentle voice within said, "And then there were three." I was tempted to look up the varied symbolic meanings of three. However, I quickly realized that I would be searching for a knowledge-based answer to my question rather than a heart-felt answer. By now, I knew that the answer was "at my finger tips."

I closed my eyes, and all of a sudden I visualized a triangle with me in the middle. A triangle is one of the most basic shapes. The triangle has three sides and three points. It holds mysteries like those of the pyramids. It is the shape that provides one of the strongest foundations. The shape is used anywhere from explaining financial security to balance of the mind, body and soul. Any child who has eaten cereal has seen the triangle on the box with an explanation of a wholesome diet. The triangle represents understanding.

I began to think of my losses: Our child, my mother and then my father. I loved and adored all three. From each passing I gained a greater understanding of love. From the loss of my child I learned how much I love as a parent. I gained compassion for all parents and families who were experiencing a child's life threatening illness or death. My mother's decline soon followed, and she passed away eight months after Cj. I lost my best confidante, my best friend, and my nurturer. I mourned and grew in compassion for all of those who have lost a mother.

After my mother's passing, I spent six months focusing on my father. We went out to lunch at least once a week. We finished conversations that we started when I was a child, but were interrupted by my marriage, child rearing (and rearing grandchildren) and my closeness to my mother. I was able to serve him after the loss of my mother and his wife of fifty-one years. I was thankful that I was really getting to know him. I was discovering the man that my mother had loved and cherished; not the man who at times argued and snapped at my mother. Suddenly he was ill and then gone. From the loss of my father I am experiencing the loss of the person whose eyes sparkled with pride when I shared my accomplishments and goals. I lost the person who stood fast to his views while allowing me to express mine. I lost the person who corrected me and through our debates expanded my views of the world. Once again I am mourning. I am quickly gaining compassion for those who have lost their fathers.

I recognize the "three" for me. I have been on a journey for many years to develop compassion and learn to serve the world by gaining knowledge through reading books. My bookshelves are so full that the rows of books are doubled. This was necessary for me. But, I now realize that I must always do the "lab work" as well. Through the books I gained knowledge. Through the lab work I gained wisdom by journaling my experience. Through the lab work I developed compassion for three aspects of mankind, because I have experienced the same significant losses. We all have a mother and a father, and many of us have a child. Most of us will or have experienced the loss of our parents, some of us the loss of a child and some of us the loss of a spouse. I gained compassion through the loss of child, mother and father.

I think my heart will hold a longing for their physical presence forever. But now when I am sad, I will imagine the "three," the triangle of father, mother and child with me in the middle. I will feel the compassion that they have for me and learn the wisdom of having compassion for myself. I have discovered that when I cry I can now say, "Today is a good day; today I am feeling." I realize that there will always be times when I am asked to do some more lab work. I have learned that when I take the time to journal and write down my experience and feelings I am rewarded with wisdom. My pain decreases while my heart expands with love and compassion. I now recognize this as my "healing." I have learned that the Healing Room is in my heart, and the key is the journal.

Epilogue

Breaking the News

062201

I went to Kaiser Hospital today for lab work. I had procrastinated for three months. My prescription was getting low, so I decided to go today before I needed to request a refill. I took the elevator to the basement and checked in with the receptionist at the lab. I asked if the order for a blood test for menopause was there; however, I was told it had expired. I mentioned that I had missed three cycles, but that they resumed after I requested the blood test. The receptionist said she also missed her menstrual cycle, and it was due to stress. She had recently lost an uncle who left a forty-five-year-old wife and five children. We talked about death, pain and the joy that can follow. She said she was glad we talked and asked to read *The Healing Room*. I promised her a copy after it was published. Then I waited forty minutes in the outside waiting room but was never called. When I finally checked with the other receptionist, she apologized and said I was supposed to have waited inside the lab room. I said, "Ah, that's right. I had forgotten. I must have needed to wait forty minutes for some reason."

Afterwards, I left the basement and accidentally pushed the button to the second floor. "Interesting," I thought. "I must need this delay also." I went back into the elevator and went to the first floor. Just before I walked out of the hospital, I noticed a gray-haired man walking in front of me. He turned, opened a door and began walking up a stairwell. My heart swelled. "It couldn't be," I thought. I called to the man's back, "Dr. Levy?" He turned and faced me. There was no recognition of me on his face, but he waited. My heart jumped into my throat and tears began to flow. "Dr. Levy, there is something I need to tell you." He knew there was something wrong. He came down to me, and I took his hand. "Do you remember your patient, Cj?" He asked for the last name. "Bohntinsky," I whispered. He remembered. My voice cracked and my eyes watered as I told him the news. I took a picture of Cj out of my wallet, and he commented on her beauty. He asked many questions. He asked if it was a long illness. I said only four months. He sighed in relief and said, "I'm glad." I shook my head and said, "For some reason you were to know about Cj's passing." Dr. Levy was on duty when Cj was born, and was her pediatrician for her first nine years. She had made many visits to him as a young child due to ear infections, severe asthma and allergies. Then Dr. Levy retired. I had never seen him since Cj's last appointment. "When did she die?" he asked gently. "On January 20, 2000," I answered. He looked straight into my eyes and said, "That is my birthday."

I told him about her strength and how she touched so many hearts. I told him about her stay at Kaiser Hospital and then at Children's Hospital. He asked if his son had been her nurse, as his son works at Children's. I said no, not that I could recall. I told him about *The Healing Room,* and he wrote down the name on the back of Cj's picture. I promised him a copy of the book. I said I planned to be speaking after the book is published. I told him about the Foundation, and he wrote down its name. I talked about how the ill children seem to be our teachers because they touch our hearts and souls and help us grow. He nodded in agreement. He of all people would know. I smiled and said, "Goodbye. I will be all right."

I walked out of the hospital and at first felt joy at the wonders of perfect timing. All the delays had led up to this meeting. Then I began to shake. My heart began to hurt and I cried. I felt like I had just re-lived Cj's whole illness and her passing. I felt like I was bearing Dr. Levy's sorrow. I felt like the sorrow of the world was upon my shoulders. "What is this all about?" I asked myself. Everything was timed perfectly so that I would see this gentle man's back and him walking up the stairs. I could have left and not said a word. I could have assumed that it was someone else. He never would have known that I had seen him. He may have never known that Cj had passed away. He would have been spared the pain and sorrow. I would have been spared this re-run of the most painful event in my life.

I felt drained the rest of the day. Even my co-workers mentioned that I seemed pensive. That evening, I told Chuck about my experience with Dr. Levy. His eyes swelled with tears. Part of me felt badly for bringing up the past even though Chuck and I often talk about Cj. However, I knew it was important for Chuck to know about the meeting. I did everything based on faith. I could have again chosen the easy way and kept it a secret, but I chose the hard way. I ignited Chuck's feelings of sorrow, which in turn ignited mine once again.

The next day Chuck and I talked about Cj. We realized that there will always be someone to whom we will need to break the news. Sometimes it will be a person from the past who

lost contact with us. As time goes on, it will be to new acquaintances. When asked if I have children I say, "Yes. We
have one on this side and one on the other." I have learned
that when I share my experience, my sorrow and my healing
I actually see gratitude on people's faces. First, I see shock
and eyes begin to glisten. Then each face brightens with a
glint of understanding, and a little bit of their burden from
fear of loss seems to lighten. Afterwards, I am rewarded with
memories that cause brief heartache and tears. I am in the
Healing Room. I once again go through the cycle of pain, sorrow, grief, tears and healing. Then I feel joy. I think we are all
in the Healing Room. The Healing Room is Life and that is
why we are here.

To Write the Author

If you wish to contact Dori Bohntinsky, please write to the author in care of In-Word Bound Publishing and we will forward your comments. Both the author and the publisher appreciate hearing from you and discovering what insights you gained from this book. In-Word Bound Publishing cannot guarantee that every letter will be answered, but all will be forwarded.

Dorothy J. Bohntinsky
c/o In-Word Bound Publishing
P.O. Box 20248
Castro Valley CA 94546

THE CJ FOUNDATION

Chuck and Dori Bohntinsky created this non-profit foundation in the memory of their daughter, Christen Jean Bohntinsky. The CJ Foundation's mission is to help lessen the anguish that families experience when faced with a life-threatening illness and/or the death of a loved one, especially a child. This mission is accomplished through charitable giving and educating the public regarding how alternative holistic therapies, in conjunction with traditional medicine, facilitate healing by reducing the negative impact of the tension and distress caused by loss.

For more information go to **http://www.CJFoundation.org** or e-mail the CJ Foundation at **cjfoundation@aol.com**